MOOD CONTROL

By the same author

THE INNOVATION MILLIONAIRES

Gene Bylinsky

MOOD CONTROL

CHARLES SCRIBNER'S SONS/NEW YORK

To my sister and my parents

LIBRARY OF CONGRESS CATALOGING IN PUBLICATION DATA

Bylinsky, Gene.
Mood control.
Includes index.
1. Psychopharmacology. I. Title.
BF207.B93 615'.788 78-929
ISBN 0-684-15586-9

This book published simultaneously in the United States of America and in Canada—Copyright under the Berne Convention

Selections from this title have appeared in *Fortune* Magazine in slightly different form.

1 3 5 7 9 11 13 15 17 19 H/C 20 18 16 14 12 10 8 6 4 2

Printed in the United States of America

Contents

Acknowledgments

Mood Control began as articles in *Fortune* magazine. Thanks are due to Robert Lubar, *Fortune*'s managing editor, for encouraging me to do the book and to Charles Whittingham, *Fortune*'s assistant publisher, for releasing the Time Inc. copyright to the *Fortune* articles that served as the bases of some of the chapters and for other kind help. I also gratefully acknowledge the assistance of many scientists who unstintingly gave of their time. Arnold J. Mandell and Alexander T. Shulgin deserve special thanks for stimulating discussions. Many thanks to Patricia Cristol for encouraging the idea of this book and shaping the outline and to Doe Coover, my editor at Scribners, for skillful editing and valuable suggestions; to Gwen and Carmela for transcribing tapes and typing portions of the manuscript, to Gregory for painstakingly preparing the index, and to Tanya for encouraging Gregory.

I would also like to express my gratitude to the following publishers and agents for permission to quote from the works cited in the text:

The Seabury Press, Inc., and Martin Secker & Warburg, for permission to quote from *The Futurological Congress* by Stanislaw Lem, English translation © 1974 the Seabury Press, Inc. Used by permission of the Seabury Press;

McIntosh and Otis, Inc., for permission to quote from *Tomorrow's Weapons* by J. H. Rothschild, Brig. Gen. USA (Ret.), McGraw-Hill Book Company, 1964. Copyright © 1964 J. H. Rothschild;

Charles C. Thomas, Publisher, for permission to quote from *Psychotropic Drugs in the Year 2000,* compiled and edited by Wayne O. Evans, Ph.D., and Nathan S. Kline, M.D., 1971. Courtesy Charles C. Thomas, Publisher, Springfield, Illinois;

Random House, Inc., for material paraphrased from *Why Your Child Is Hyperactive,* by Ben F. Feingold, M.D., © 1974;

J. B. Lippincott Company, for a quotation from Charles Dickens's *A Christmas Carol,* illustrated by Arthur Rackham, 1952;

Stein & Day Publishers and McIntosh and Otis, Inc., for a brief summary from the book *Psychodietetics,* copyright © 1974 E. Cheraskin, W. M. Ringsdorf, Jr., with Arlene Brecher. Reprinted with permission of Stein & Day Publishers and McIntosh and Otis, Inc.;

Harper & Row, Publishers, for permission to use a quotation from *Violence and the Brain* by Vernon H. Mark and Frank R. Ervin.

PART I

The Coming Psychem Supermarket

CHAPTER ONE

A New Class of Users

I finally learned how to come into possession of an encyclopedia. I already own one now—the whole thing contained in three glass vials. Bought them in a science psychedeli. Books are no longer read but eaten, not made of paper but of some informational substance; fully digestible, sugar-coated. I also did a little browsing in a psychem supermarket. Self-service. Arranged on the shelves are beautifully-packaged low-calorie opinionates, gullibloons—credibility beans? —abstract extract in antique gallon jugs, and iffies, argumunchies, puritands and dyecstasy chips.

The imaginative Polish science fiction writer Stanislaw Lem wrote the above passage in his book *The Futurological Congress,* just six years ago. Lem's fictitious "psychem" (psychiatric chemistry) society is a utopia based on a "chemocratic" system of government wherein whatever people want, they get—helped by strong doses of mood- and mind-influencing drugs. There are both "benignmizers" such as Hedonidol, Euphoril, Inebrium, Felicitine, Ecstasine, and Halcyonal and their antagonists, Furiol, Rabiditine, Dementium, Flagellan, and Juggernol. Vigilax disperses all states of somnolence, trances, illusions, figments, and nightmares. Obliterine and Amnesol purge the mind of unpleasant memories, and Authentium creates synthetic recollections of things that never happened. Duetine doubles a person's consciousness in such a way that "you can hold discussions with yourself, on any topic (determined by a separate drug)." Children learn reading and writing from orthographic sodas. Optimistizine and Seraphinol put people in the best possible humor. A few drops of Credendium make one person applaud another's every word; dehallucinides create an illusion that there is no illusion. Business letters with gentle reminders about accounts outstanding and amounts owed are saturated with a volatile substance that awakens the debtor's scruples and sense of responsibility.

So fast is drug technology moving these days that the kind of chemical behavior modification envisioned by Lem is not that far from reality. "We are on the edge of a choose-your-mood society," says one scientist. "Those of us who work in this field see a developing potential for nearly total control of human emotional status, mental functioning, and will to act. These human phenomena can be started, stopped, or eliminated by the use of various types of chemical substances."

Scientists exploring the brain, that endlessly complex organ, have just recently begun to discover chemical signals of specific fractions of behavior. One such chemical enhances visual attention not only in the mentally retarded but also in normal people. Moreover, it promises to increase motivation and to improve failing memory in the elderly. Another newly discovered brain chemical makes people forget unpleasant experiences, just like Lem's science-fictional Obliterine and Amnesol. A third restores sexual potency in males and allows previously infertile women to have children (see Chapter 2).

Side by side with these discoveries, a separate but closely related area of research beginning to produce results is the synthesis of new mind- and mood-influencing drugs, chemically akin to LSD, mescaline, and other psychedelic, or mind-opening, agents. In a radical departure from the usual approach to drug design, intended to help people who are identifiably sick, these new drugs promise to help *normal* people in many different ways, from improving their creative capabilities to easing the pain of divorce to producing exhilarating effects similar to those of alcohol but without liquor's caloric content or damage to the liver.

These new drugs go beyond the familiar amphetamine pep pills and barbiturate thrill pills discovered long ago by a multitude of users ranging from suburban housewives trying to stay slim and cope with household chores to long-distance truck drivers on demanding schedules to college students cramming for exams. The new drugs are much more specific in what they do. Whereas amphetamine pep pills, for instance, encourage a person to do more of the same repetitive tasks (during World War II the Japanese gave amphetamine tablets to their war factory workers), the new drugs are capable of enhancing and suppressing specific moods and emotions such as attention, intention, anger, fear, and joy. In often startling new research that is still unknown to the public, scientists are discovering that they can play the mood-and-emotion keyboard much as a pianist plays notes and chords.

They are also making surprising findings that what we eat may have a lot to do with how we act, because the brain chemicals that govern behavior are built up from substances in our food. True choose-your-mood diets aren't far away (see Chapter 3).

This emerging ability to extend the range of behavior and emotions opens up a myriad of possibilities. In benign hands, these new capabilities can improve man's creative and productive capacities and free him of unnecessary worries and anxieties. In sinister hands, they can be turned into a weapon as potent, though much less conspicuous, as the atom bomb.

Not surprisingly, military planners were among the first large-scale users of the mind-influencing drugs. They began thinking about employing mind-altering drugs such as LSD as weapons of war not long after their appearance. In the early 1950s the Central Intelligence Agency and the U.S. military became greatly concerned that the Soviet secret police, the KGB, had leaped ahead in the use of hallucinogens and related psychochemicals. First there were bizarre confessions by Hungarian Cardinal Mindszenty apparently obtained under the influence of truth-serumlike drugs.* Then there were intelligence reports about extremely active Soviet research in the field. On top of that, Communist governments suddenly began buying abroad possible hal-

*There is reason to believe that Soviet use of mind-influencing drugs on political prisoners goes as far back as the great purges of the 1930s. When the Germans overran Soviet Crimea in World War II, they discovered an experimental garden where Soviet researchers had been experimenting with exotic plants that yield, among other things, a speech-inducing drug. This drug, harmaline, derived from a plant called *Peganum harmala,* was combined with an extract from another plant, *Annabis affala.* Russian gardeners still in the Crimea told the Germans that harmaline had been used as a speech inducer at the show trials. The compound produces a posthypnotic effect under which the person drugged repeats exactly what is suggested to him. Harmaline is also found in a South American rain forest climbing vine. It has been used as an ingredient of a sacred Amazon Indian drink employed in initiating shamans and inducing a state of clairvoyance.

lucinogenic drugs in large quantities. Most ominous of all, the CIA and its western counterparts began to capture KGB agents carrying syringes of fluid designed to ease control of people they had planned to kidnap.

This information indicated that a major portion of American forces could be rendered helpless and defenseless by drugs that were odorless, colorless, and tasteless. There was also a threat that our most sensitive security matters could be unknowingly compromised. Most of all, U.S. military and intelligence authorities feared that an alternative to the atom bomb was about to emerge, a weapon that might render large forces helpless—though only temporarily—and without any permanent damage to those forces or their surroundings. A country might thus be overrun without anyone's being killed.

To meet the anticipated threat, U.S. agencies in 1955 initiated a program that had three specific objectives. First, it sought to determine which hallucinogenic drugs might provide an effective alternative to more drastic weaponry. Second, it wanted to ascertain the possible uses of such drugs in intelligence operations—a speech-inducing drug that would untie the tongues of uncooperative captured enemy agents was of particular interest, for instance.* Finally, the military and the CIA

*The earlier "truth serums" widely publicized in this country in the 1950s were misnomers in almost every sense. Although administered by injection, these derivatives of barbiturates, sodium pentathol and sodium amytol, were not serums, which are blood fluids. The alleged ability of truth serums to elicit truth was almost equally mislabeled. These drugs transport a person into the twilight zone of altered consciousness, where the drug taker becomes dependent on the drug giver. In this state some persons can be induced to tell the truth they were formerly withholding, but others are inspired to say what the drug giver wants to hear. People with a strong sense of identity generally can defeat the compulsion to change their story, whereas those with weaker wills, and persons inclined toward depression and feelings of guilt, are likely to crack under drug influence or at least to change their stories to accommodate the interrogators. Under the influence of such drugs, some American prisoners in Korea capitulated to their captors and changed their stories, but others told their inquisitors what they thought they wanted to hear. Defense lawyers in this country were quick to cash in on the "truth serums" to try to prove the innocence of their clients. Although reversals of death sentences were obtained on this basis, many drug experts felt that such evidence should have been ruled inadmissible in view of the uncertain effects of the drugs.

"Truth serums" were employed with success in clinical settings on occasion. In 1963 were eager to develop an antidote to such drugs, should they be used against U.S. or Allied forces or civilians.

The military and the CIA entered into research contracts with universities and independent institutes and also began their own testing. Early on, it became clear that the hallucinogens packed a potent punch—a potential invisible weapon to muddle the mind. In one fairly large-scale test, for example, troops exposed to one of these psychochemicals were not even conscious of their abnormal condition, which was so pronounced that they were unable to follow simple commands and perform normal tasks with acceptable accuracy. Only an outsider not exposed to the drug and coming upon the confused soldiers could recognize their behavior as eccentric.

In all, about fifteen hundred men received LSD and other hallucinogens in army tests and untold hundreds of others in CIA-sponsored research. (How the CIA-military program got trapped in a dangerous cul-de-sac of the ethics and morality of using such drugs on unwitting subjects is told in the Epilogue.)

Although the CIA and the military understandably have not been very communicative about their conclusions and what drugs they considered promising, work on psychochemicals continues. One outgrowth of this work has been the development of BZ (3-quinuclidinyl benzilate), a powerful psychochemical that causes both physical and mental incapacitation. It starts with a feeling of dryness in the mouth and goes on to blur the vision and produce a stumbling gait, loss of memory, urine retention, and, finally, total immobility. Inadvertently, soldiers continue to be exposed to the drug, as this 1977 news item indicates.

---

the Civil Aeronautics Administration elicited details of an air crash from a seriously injured physician who had been aboard the plane. Before taking the drug the doctor could recall only the general activities preceding the crash. The serums were also successfully administered to help some victims of amnesia recover their memory. But as elicitors of truth in people who had made up their minds to lie, or in people who believed their fantasies, the drugs usually failed to work, and their use therefore declined sharply after the mid 1960s. A much more successful "truth" drug is alcohol since, as everyone knows, when present at certain levels in the blood it "loosens" tongues.

G.I.'s Hallucinogen to Be Studied

DUGWAY, Utah, Jan. 30 (UPI)—Experts in the disposal of chemical warfare weapons will arrive at Dugway Proving Grounds tomorrow to investigate how a soldier was accidentally exposed to the hallucinogenic agent BZ. The incident left Specialist 5 Ronald Mutchko hospitalized with hallucinations and rapid heartbeat. He became exposed to the agent Thursday while he and another soldier were opening cluster bombs containing the BZ.

How hallucinogens and other psychochemicals might be used in wartime isn't hard to imagine. Brig. Gen. J. H. Rothschild, commanding general of the U.S. Army Chemical Corps Research and Development Command, wrote following his retirement: "Think of the effect of using this type of material covertly on a higher headquarters of a military unit, or overtly a large organization. . . . It's easy to foresee that a military commander under the effects of LSD-25 would lose his ability to make logical, rational decisions and issue coherent orders. Group cooperation would fall apart."*

As for uses against enemy civilians, Rothschild spoke of the obvious possibility of incorporating psychochemical agents into food, drugs, and even cosmetics. The main limitation on the variety of methods that can be employed is the knowledge and imagination of the user. Little wonder that scientists have concluded that psychochemicals will be the most difficult of all weaponry to control and supervise if disarmament ever comes.

Always a step ahead of conventional planners, Stanislaw Lem visualized a more positive and more amusing "psychem" weapon he called cryptobellina. Applied as an aerosol, it led to universal disarmament by creating in soldiers on both sides an irresistible urge to run out, find some rope, and tie themselves up.

Military applications aside, there are disturbing possibilities of malevolent or misguided use of the new mind drugs to harm or control people. There will almost certainly be widespread abuse of these drugs. When they become generally known, we will probably see a tremendous demand from a new class of drug users—law-abiding citizens who

*J. H. Rothschild, Brig. Gen. USA (Ret), *Tomorrow's Weapons, Chemical and Biological* (New York: McGraw-Hill Book Company, 1964).

will want to enhance their creative, sexual, and other potentials.

Since no mechanism exists today for legal introduction and controlled use of mind medications, they will be illegally manufactured and sold on the black market. The most sought-after of them will undoubtedly command very high prices. "The real problem in the field of psychopharmaceuticals," says Nathan S. Kline, a pioneer in the field, "is not so much the creation of new classes of drugs, but determining who shall make the decisions as to when they should be used, on whom, and by whom."

These unresolved questions have taken on a certain urgency because, whether we like it or not, the capability of synthesizing highly specific mood- and mind-influencing drugs is already here.

Man has, of course, sought (and employed) mind-expanding drugs for thousands of years. Although Indians in the New World appear to have discovered most of the hallucinogenic drugs in plant sources, such as the various hallucinogenic so-called sacred mushrooms, the denizens of the Old World and their descendants in America weren't that far behind. They, too, employed "magic" plant extracts, such as the belladonna compounds used in witchcraft. The Old World compounds are more properly termed *delusinogens* than hallucinogens, because they produce delusions rather than illusions, but they can be as potent as the hallucinogens. Some researchers think, for instance, that the Salem witch trials were the result of a massive poisoning with rye bread contaminated with an ergot fungus containing a hallucinogen similar to LSD that caused bizarre, nightmarish visions in the normally placid Puritans.

Modern-day possibilities, however, didn't really hit drug designers until recent decades of deliberate, massive use of mind-influencing drugs that pointed to the possibilities of manipulating the nuances of human behavior.

Early hints of where mood control was going came from observation by psychiatrists treating patients suffering from mania, depression, and other manifestations of mental problems with psychopharmacological agents. The psychiatrists noticed that the antipsychotic drugs had powerful effects on many aspects of their patients' personalities, far beyond the major symptoms that called for the drug treatment in the first place. They could see how previously quiet patients on the so-called tricyclic antidepressants would suddenly become impersonally talkative. One psychiatrist recalled a mousy forty-seven-year-old spinster suddenly telling him he was late for an appointment and demanding an explanation. They could see also how amphetamines organized the thinking of some people and how ruthless and aggressive men suddenly acquired a certain tenderness after exposure to small doses of hallucinogens. Bullies suddenly began thinking of children and baby animals frolicking in the grass.

It was the exposure to hallucinogens such as LSD and mescaline that offered the most intriguing possibilities of all. A whole generation of youngsters, whose often mindless use of psychedelic drugs sent them on mind-bending journeys into unreal worlds, could now be observed. Eloquent pioneers such as Aldous Huxley had explored edges of those worlds earlier, but never had so many Westerners traveled so far with the help of drugs and brought back so many fantastic tales.

Psychedelic drugs, such as LSD, psilocybin, and psilocin (from mushrooms such as *Psilocybe mexicana* and *Stropharia cubensis*), and mescaline, which comes from the peyote cactus, are in a class by themselves. They are unlike sedatives such as barbiturates, stimulants such as amphetamines, or tranquilizers such as Librium or Miltown. They are also not like narcotic drugs such as the opiates, which are addictive. A percentage of amphetamine and barbiturate users become abusers. Psychedelic drugs are not physically addictive, and, of course, they produce psychological experiences spectacularly different from the other mind-influencing drugs.

Among these experiences are fascinating changes in perception. Sounds are transformed into visual sensations, each tone or noise producing a kaleidoscopic color picture. Objects such as flowers or stones appear to pulsate and come to life. Incredible scenes are imagined with one's eyes closed. Incidents from the past are relived. Time and space are transcended. Many users also claim that their artistic perceptions —appreciation of music and painting—are enhanced.

But no one has produced any artistic masterpieces under the influence of hallucinogens, and the drugs often have adverse side effects. A sense of unmanageability, even panic, on occasion grip LSD and mescaline users. In others, anxiety or visual aberrations persist for days after use.

A healthy shift away from the often dangerous use of hallucinogenic drugs is now in the making as careful investigators pursue in their laboratories the question of how derivatives of the powerful mind-influencing drugs can be made to work for the benefit of man without harmful hallucinogenic and other side effects. "There is a new realm," says Arnold J. Mandell, cochairman of the department of psychiatry at the University of California at San Diego. "I think the era of the new brain drugs will fractionate out aspects of behavior that we never paid any attention to before."

Mandell notes as an example that attachment as a human phenomenon is traceable as a brain system. One of the commonly used antidepressant drug families, the tricyclic antidepressants, in addition to removing depression in most people also thins out the dependence patients have on their spouses and children. When a user of this drug anticipates the loss of a loved one somehow—such as through divorce—he doesn't experience the separation anxiety as painfully as he normally would. We can also see that the function of attachment must be chemically modulated in the brain by observing animals. Cats, for instance, aren't as attached to man as dogs are, presumably because cats' brain chemistry is somewhat different. Scientists predict that when the biochemistry of behavior is deciphered it will be possible to assign specific emotions and actions to the presence or absence of specific chemicals in the brain—a dramatic shift from the environmental psychiatry that has ruled us for so long.

These advances stem from the often startling new knowledge about the brain. The old view represented the brain as a lightning-fast but rather rigid electrical switchboard, "an enchanted loom, with millions of flashing shuttles," as one scientist described it.

In the new view the brain is a much more complex, more interesting organ. It looks much more like an enchanted forest instead of an enchanted loom. It's a place where dendrites, the antennae of the neurons, constantly grow out of neuronal bodies like interweaving branches of giant trees, where neighboring neurons whisper to each other at energy levels so low that they are hardly measurable, and where cells called glia—in which the neurons are embedded—move about, influencing the activity of the neurons. The brain is changing, remodeling, and restructuring itself from instant to instant.

The great recent discovery has been that the biggest changes in the brain are directed by chemical substances acting in conjunction with electrical signals. Thus, the brain was found to be not only an electrical computer but a computer submerged in a chemical cauldron where chemicals of different shades and hues can light up or darken the enchanted forest.

The brain responds instantaneously to millions of electrical impulses that constantly pour into it from sensory receptors. A thought can, of course, set off these impulses just as efficiently as a sight can. The signals are processed with lightning speed and coded into computerlike yes or no commands. The impulses then speed along the remarkable network that consists of neurons. A neuron is shaped somewhat like a tree, with the cell body at the top. From there branch out the dendrites, which receive messages from neighboring neurons. The tree's trunk is the axon, the neuron's transmission cable. Its length can be impressive. In man, for instance, axons that connect the big toe to the spinal cord can be three feet long. In a giraffe they may be twelve feet long.

Millions of axons run down the spinal column like coaxial cables. A signal transmitted down the axon is bioelectrical until it comes to a synapse, one of the hundreds of the axon's tiny junction points that connect with other neurons. The synapse is a slit less than a millionth of an inch wide. The current in the axon is too weak to bridge this gap, so instead it activates transmitter chemicals located in storage granules at nerve endings. The chemical substances enter the gap and activate the neighboring neuron at its receptor sites with a replica of the original impulse. When the signal reaches its destination, such as a muscle, the signal produces the desired action or movement. When the signal acts on neurons in a certain region of the brain—a pathway of a particular mood—it calls forth an emotion or a behavioral act.

These natural chemical messengers of behavior are known as neurotransmitters. In the mid-1950s, manipulation of the neurotransmitter levels in the brain with psychotropic (mind-influencing) drugs that resembled neurotransmitters in structure—antidepressants, neuroleptics, stimulants—dramatically reduced the population of mental hospitals (see Chapter 4).

By using psychotropic drugs to illuminate the pathways of emotion and psychiatric disease, scientists have traced networks of neurons that respond to specific neurotransmitters. Of particular interest have been the so-called biogenic amines, derivatives of amino acids. Among the most important of these amines are dopamine, norepinephrine (or noradrenaline), and serotonin.

Loss of dopamine from the part of the brain called the basal ganglia is what causes the disorganized muscle activity of Parkinson's disease and possibly the disordered thought patterns of schizophrenia. Norepinephrine influences a wide range of functions through a diffuse network of neurons. Depression appears to be related to a deficiency of norepinephrine at certain synapses, and manic states to an excess of the same neurotransmitter.

Changes in serotonin levels in the brain alter an organism's ability to evaluate the contextual cues of its environment. The alterations influence many types of behavior. There are hints that some people who commit suicide are suffering from a serotonin deficit.

How can a subjective feeling be explained in terms of how neurons act? What is it that the biogenic amines do exactly to influence a person's mood?

Seymour Kety, who served as the first scientific director of the National Institute of Mental Health and now directs psychiatric research laboratories at the Massachusetts General Hospital in Boston, offers some intriguing thoughts on the biological underpinnings of moods.

We haven't really appreciated the importance of the value system to the brain. Over a billion years of evolution, it is easy to conceive that the species would have learned and genetically endowed each individual with a means of evaluating results of behavior as good or bad. Animals would have learned through evolution that food is good because food leads to survival. That sexual activity is good because any animal that didn't think so would die out fairly soon. On the other hand, destruction of tissue would be bad. Hunger would be bad. These are values in terms of survival of the species, and species that didn't incorporate these values would die out. Now the problem is, how do these values get translated into everyday experience?

I like to think that the biogenic amines are the systems that mediate between these values, and that moods are the subjective counterparts of the biological processes by which various new experiences are evaluated, coded, and stored with an appropriate value—good or bad. It is not by accident that with the things that are good for the species, we have pleasure; and with things that are bad for the species we have pain. It's conceivable that with pleasure you have one kind of profile of chemical substances released in the brain, and with pain you have another kind of profile in a kind of color coding. One amine may be related to one value and another amine to another value. Perhaps the way in which these two amines are mixed together could give you various shades between extreme good and extreme bad. Somehow I have a feeling that noradrenaline and serotonin may have some relationship to what is good and bad—to the value system in the brain.

In his inimitable fashion, Stanislaw Lem presents this same idea: "All perception is but a change in the concentration of hydrogen ions on the surface of the brain cells. Seeing me, you actually experience a disturbance in the sodium-potassium equilibrium across your neuron membranes. So all we have to do is to send a few well-chosen molecules down into those cortical mitochondria, activate the right neurohumoral-synaptic transmission sites, and your fondest dreams come true."

Lem's fantasy comes pretty close to reality, for psychedelic drugs resemble natural neurotransmitters and can be used to manipulate moods and emotions. LSD and a number of similar drugs all have an indole ring, a basic structural unit that also appears in serotonin. Mescaline is closely related to the natural catecholamines norepinephrine and epinephrine (adrenalin). The drugs interact with their analogous neurotransmitters, stimulating or inhibiting their activity at the synapses. For example, LSD and related drugs, chemical cousins of serotonin, appear to inhibit the utilization of serotonin in certain areas of the brain, releasing it from serotonin-imposed inhibitions.

Arnold Mandell, a pioneer tester of the new drugs and a brilliant biochemical psychiatrist to whom we owe many of our new insights into the mind, believes that the new emotion-enhancing and behavior-improving agents act by holding down man's ancient and primitive "reptilian" brain while bringing out the best in the new cortex. A crocodile's or a frog's mere knob of a brain typify the reptilian brain's limitations. This brain, the antecedents of which go back perhaps 200 million years, is located mainly in the brain stem and controls such basic instinctual mechanisms as courting, mating, and selecting home-sites. It also controls such reflex activities of the body as muscular motion and glandular function, the flow of blood and the beat of the heart.

Mammals developed an increasingly more elaborate mesolimbic, or middle, brain that encloses the old reptile within us. The middle brain controls the senses of smell and taste, supervises activities inside the body, and directs emotions.

On top of the middle brain is man's upper brain, the neocortex, which makes man unique. It allows abstract thinking, anticipation, problem solving, writing, and speech.

Mandell vividly describes the haunting contrast between these different levels of the human mind.

> The reptilian brain, when aroused, when allowed to express itself, is aggressive, competitive, suspicious, angry, bound by territorial limits, and insensitive to new input. It's the brain of the groin psychologists—Freud, Darwin, and Marx. It's the brain that controls the settling of a country, the establishment of the army, establishing dominance over that country. It's the cultural deification of the Marines, of macho and of pro football. It's the killer brain whose ecstasy is winning—a triumph which may involve the humiliation of others.
>
> The other, newer system in the brain we visualize more in terms of perceptual arousal. It is not bound by territory but is free to float. It is sensitive to new input. It is much more interested in beauty than triumph. The ecstasy of that system is insight or discovery.

The split between mood-influenced beliefs and rational thinking embedded in our heads has intrigued some of the world's best minds.

Arthur Koestler described the situation to a conference on future psychotropic drugs.

> There seems to be an icebox built somewhere into our skulls which is the seat of cold logic and rational thought, and next to it there is a hothouse of irrational, mood-based beliefs. But the two don't interact, there is no integration. Instead of integration, there is a kind of a chronic, schizophrenic split, on the psychological level, between emotion and reason, faith and logic, and underlying it on the psychological level, a "schizophysiology." In the last stages of our evolution, the neocortex developed at such a rapid and explosive rate that it never became completely integrated with the phylogenetically older parts of the brain. The result seems to be inadequate coordination, or insufficient feedback between the modern brain, as the seat of the language or rational and abstract thought on the one hand, and the archaic parts which mediate emotional behavior. This theory provides a very plausible evolutionary explanation of what has gone wrong with our species. And if this diagnosis of the predicament is correct, then there is some hope that neuropsychopharmacology might find an answer to it.

One of the most imaginative answer seekers, Mandell, with an independent California drug designer, Alexander T. Shulgin, has been investigating such intriguing questions as whether creativity can be enhanced with derivatives of the hallucinogenic drugs. In his drugs Shulgin combines some of the chemical features of mescaline with a side chain of amphetamine. A highly intuitive man, Shulgin has come up with some psychopharmacological bombshells. "A number of materials I have been working on," he says, "are amplifiers of specific senses that will enhance the visual, the interpretive color sense, or the auditory acuity, without blanketing the entire body with intoxication and confusion."

Whereas amphetamine typically strengthens the fixed patterns of response that characterize the reptilian brain—a student on amphetamine once happily counted cornflakes all night in a lab—Shulgin's drugs release the creative part of the brain from serotonin-imposed inhibition. The new drugs are effective in much lower doses than hallucinogens such as LSD and mescaline, and they can be administered in a wide range of doses without inducing hallucinations and the frightening dissolution of individuality that LSD can cause.

LSD doses are measured in millionths of a gram. An amount of LSD equal to an aspirin tablet is enough to produce effects in three thousand people.

An intense man with a leonine mane of prematurely gray hair, Shulgin began to design his remarkable drugs more than a decade ago. He is a Ph.D. pharmacologist who had worked for a big chemical company. On his own, he soon began to devise drugs with such specific action that his skills amazed psychiatrists.

His early drugs had to be tested behind the scenes. Testing such experimental drugs on human volunteers is easier abroad than in this country, so Shulgin supplied some of his early drugs to Claudio Naranjo, a psychiatrist at the University of Chile. Testing one early Shulgin drug on student volunteers, Naranjo found that the students' thinking and emotions were enhanced, without the perceptual distortions of hallucinogens. Hallucinogens depersonalize a drug taker (he often feels a sense of oneness with the universe), but Shulgin's drugs intensify a person's awareness of self without loss of contact with the environment or distortions in thinking.

Enhancement of creativity with the new drugs is one of the exciting areas being explored by Shulgin and Mandell. On the face of it, creativity would appear to be one of the most complex human functions, but it turns out that it is one of the most easily stimulated. Shulgin's compounds produce a feeling of newness or novelty in an old situation. Rats tested for habituation (in this instance their ability to get used to air puffs blown at them by a special device) react to each puff as if it were the first.

Tested on students, one Shulgin drug produced a striking improvement in their writing ability. Although amphetamine increases the amount of writing, it usually becomes vacuous and repetitious. "When you give a Shulgin compound," says Mandell, "the writing will be long but it will have beauty and detail."

Shulgin is working with the part of the mescaline molecule that produces inhibition of habituation, or stops a person from getting used to familiar things. A Shulgin drug called DOET makes the subjects relaxed and receptive to new ideas without hallucinogenic effects. Recalled a student volunteer who took a series of tests after ingesting a small dose of DOET: "I was quite aware that I was being impatient with the tests, but I still wanted to do well. I was consciously trying not to rush through just to get it done, whereas if I had taken LSD, I would have just said to hell with everything."

Others found DOET to heighten their sense of taste. "The almonds were really supertasty—I couldn't believe when I tasted one," said a student. Another added, "I could close my eyes and create very vividly any sorts of images that I wanted to." Still another recalled that he cried with joy when listening to music with his eyes closed.

A number of sophisticated social scientists, including anthropologists and psychiatrists, who have taken Shulgin compounds have described several kinds of enhancement they experienced: new insights, attention to previously unnoticed aspects of a situation, perception of new problem-solving possibilities, and a marked gain in creative capacity. People have tried to solve problems under the influence of LSD and other hallucinogens, of course. But those drugs are such commanding mistresses in their own right that their users soon get distracted by the drugs' effects.

Interestingly, Shulgin himself has gained new insights into drug design by taking his own creativity drugs.

> It's difficult to describe what happens when you take a creativity drug, because it's not explicitly stateable in twenty-five words. When you address yourself to a problem under the influence of a drug, you take hold of the problem by the lower-left-hand corner so to speak—where you have never taken hold of it before. You find it's not a direct approach to a problem. It's almost like a derivative approach *to* the approach of solving the problem. You begin to analyze the reasons why you have a hangup. Rather than approach the problem in the classic way you already had, you find that your reasons for approaching the problem are often more important than the reasons for solving it. And suddenly you have an oblique view on what you have been working with and you find a crevice or a little spot that is extremely productive and effective. This has often happened to me in connection with chemical problems. Which brings the whole thing into an interesting paradox—a kind of a bootstrap operation.

Suddenly Shulgin will get a new view of the molecular structure he is working on at the time. Creativity drugs direct his brain to visualize the chemistry problem in terms of symbols that are not the usual chemical formulas but represent the structure of the molecule he is working on. "It's as though you had a neurological capability wired into the brain—something that Ma Bell had tucked away in her computer and you just have no way of dialing in because the neurotransmitters are not at hand, they are not mobilized, they are suppressed, or something is amiss. The drug catalyzes it."

Of course, these drugs don't make a clod suddenly creative. Shulgin tried them on a small group of not particularly creative people and failed to get any response. "You are not seeing the emergence of creativity *de novo,*" he says, "but you are allowing its organization in a person who should and could have it organized but does not because of a blockage or intuitive blindness. You can't design a pill that will write a play in a man's head." Adds Mandell, "When you recreate the first-time freshness in an old, experienced hand, then you've got creativity."

The finding that dullards cannot be made creative with drugs is in keeping with the discoveries of modern neuroanatomy that the brain is tied together as a network and that a person uses all of his brain. "The old mythology that human beings are using only some percentage of the brain is nonsense," says Gary Lynch, a young neurophysiologist at the University of California's Irvine campus. "A chimpanzee—whose brain most closely resembles man's—is not going to learn to read, and there is no drug on earth, I think, that will do that."

But there are distinct chemistries underlying attention and intention, separation and loss, mastery and coping, and such components of behavior can be influenced with drugs. Moving in this direction, Shulgin has synthesized a new kind of antidepressant. Unlike commonly used antidepressants, Shulgin's compound, a variant of mescaline, is not a stimulant to normal people. "But in a person who is demotivated, acting below his usual capacity," Shulgin says, "the drug brings that person back to his normal motivation." The compound is in the final stages of testing by a big drug company and has a good chance of becoming a commercial antidepressant.

Shulgin calls another of his drugs a low-calorie martini. In designing it he tried to duplicate the exhilarating effects of the first or second drink—and stop there. He thinks he has succeeded with a drug that acts in about fifteen minutes and whose relaxing effects last an hour or two. The drug has no caloric value and none of alcohol's damaging effect on the liver. Shulgin describes the effects he has tried to create:

In drinking, there is this marvelous level, somewhere during the second martini, you can't say what's happening but suddenly everything is a little bit more brighter, conversation is a little bit more relaxed, the music is suddenly proper, you are fitting into the environment. That's the goal of alcohol drinking. I find it an absolutely fabulous moment. I've tried to define the beginning and the end of it, because it doesn't take much more alcohol when that moment is lost. You continue drinking for the purpose of maintaining it, but when you do, you're wiped out. You get into that third drink, and fourth drink, and the next thing you know, you've tripped over something, your motor reactions are disappearing, intellectually you're getting sloppy, your speech is going, and the next thing you know you're into dinner and wine and it gets noisy, and you've lost that magic period. For some people it's longer, for others shorter. One of the targets I had was to develop a drug that would induce this sensory amplification period—this slightly altered consciousness—that would build up the effect in twenty to thirty minutes and dissipate within an hour and a half. I found a drug that almost precisely meets these requirements.

It causes a distinct awareness in the early stages—oh, I felt that drink—is the first thought that comes across your mind. Whatever occurs to a person who had an alcoholic drink at that point is occurring to the person who takes this drug—a disinhibition of some sensory constraint that allows a person to suddenly not quite get lightheaded but to be able to act as if he were lightheaded. He cries a little bit, laughs a little bit, he is a little bit more honest in his responses. In alcohol, this very quickly turns into sloppiness. With the drug, it works into yet more of the same (lightheadedness). But I think it's really a virtue over alcohol. The people who get through the one-and-a-half martini stage expect to get sloppy, to have a refill poured down their pants' leg—these are patterns they've learned through years of use. They are part of the intoxication process. This doesn't hold true of the drug. It's not the continuation of the intoxication stage but a change in a new direction. I think an ideal alcoholic cocktail would be one that would bring you into that one-and-a-half martini stage and lock you right there.

In designing such specificity into drugs, Shulgin takes advantage of emerging skills in extra-fine modification of molecular structures. It has become clear that extremely small changes in molecular structure can cause dramatically wide shifts in biological action. Shulgin's antidepressant, for instance, differs by a single carbon atom from STP, a powerful hallucinogen that he synthesized and which is about one hundred times more powerful than mescaline. (Sometimes, of course, Shulgin misses. One of his drugs, as an unplanned side effect, causes auditory distortion. A slightly out-of-tune piano sounds so bad to the drug taker that it becomes unplayable. And to his ears a normally high voice drops to basso.)

Drug designers are beginning to tailor drugs to the tiny receptors on the surfaces of cells. A receptor accepts specific substances that have structures that fit a receptor's particular shape. These structures cause the receptor to transmit an appropriate signal into the interior of the cell. A search is on for receptors for all sorts of feelings, emotions, and aspects of behavior. Drugs can then be designed to fit the particular receptors, either to evoke the desired behavior or to block undesirable behavior. Says Shulgin, "The time will come when we'll separate all our senses and capabilities—the visual from the auditory, the tactile from the sense of smell as well as wit, intellectual capability, creativity—and enhance them with drugs."

Application of the new mind drugs so far is just a small beginning. Mandell and others see a legitimate use for the new drugs to ease the pain of separation or divorce, to allow people dying prematurely from incurable diseases to face death with equanimity, even to eliminate an employee's fear of the boss. "Objections to such boosts in emotion or behavior," says Mandell, "could only come from people who feel that medicine must taste bad to do good."

To this list of applications Nathan Kline, a pioneering psychopharmacologist and director of the Rockland, New York, State Hospital, adds some other intriguing possibilities: prolonging childhood so as to increase acquisition of knowledge and skills; reducing or even circumventing the need for sleep; provoking or relieving guilt to treat criminals, among others; shortening or extending experienced time to enhance appreciation of music, for instance, and, conversely, to speed up the passage of undesirable events.

How soon such drugs will be made available legally is another question. "There is no social, scientific, or medical apparatus for optimizing normal human behavior," says Mandell. "I think it will take decades because there is no aegis in our society for introduction of performance or life-improving drugs. Under whose aegis could we administer a creativity drug, for instance? It isn't that you're sick, so no doctor can give it to you. There is a wall against all this work."

A strange dichotomy that exists in social customs could be a serious barrier to the introduction of mood-control medications. There is a widespread belief, for instance, that use of drugs in a social setting is bad. On the other hand, use of alcohol in such a setting is considered proper. In drug use a lone-wolf user is tolerated for his idiosyncrasies, but a lone-wolf alcoholic is frowned upon.

It's not that scientists such as Mandell and Shulgin advocate a Brave New World society *à la* Huxley or Lem. (Huxley's drug in *Brave New World* was soma: "One cubic centimeter cures ten gloomy sentiments.") In contrast, Mandell and Shulgin see use of the new mind drugs as being only episodic, say, by busy people who don't have time to exercise or run; those forms of exercise can automatically induce some of the euphoric effects produced by drugs. They argue, though, that research should be pursued if for no other reason than to head off the appearance of illicit drugs in this field, which may have dangerous side effects.

To find ways to minimize or eliminate the hazards and to identify and develop the constructive potential of these powerful agents would be a worthwhile task. The alternatives are not attractive. Sooner than anyone suspects, the lack of a mechanism to introduce such drugs might create difficulties for society whose dimensions will make the mind drug revolution we've already gone through seem like a minor conflagration by comparison.

CHAPTER TWO

Peptides: The Ultimate Aphrodisiacs (among Other Things)

I can see someone like Woody Allen coming into a party with a nasal spray and going "tchee, tchee, tchee." And people start undressing. I can also see another possibility. You have a patient and you give him this drug. He goes out and rapes a girl. Who is morally responsible? The implications of this research have not even been considered.

The scientist who drew that vignette wasn't daydreaming but was describing, rather, some real-life possibilities now arising thanks to the discovery that a hormone made in the brain and acting on it could be the ultimate aphrodisiac. In trail-blazing but still little-known research, the hormone has already been used with great success to restore sexual potency in impotent males and to induce ovulation and successful pregnancy in women never before able to have children.

The name of this substance is Luteinizing Releasing Hormone, or LRH for short. The implications of its discovery are staggering, of course. Who would control the distribution of this new aphrodisiac or of a countermanding agent, an antagonist that blocks sexual function and desire? Analogues, or chemical copies hundreds of times more potent than natural LRH, have already been developed (reducing the cost of a single dose from one hundred dollars to a few cents), as have the antagonists that block its action.

Although LRH use is being carefully supervised at the research institutions involved, there is no guarantee that it and its antagonists are not going to be made illegally or secretly in the future, or be stolen from legitimate suppliers. Already, LRH is being marketed in Europe for diagnostic purposes and U.S. drug companies are investigating its manufacture.

Countries and individuals could employ the hormone as a subtle yet extremely powerful weapon. One can easily visualize one country waging a secret sex subversion war on another by slipping LRH antagonists into drinking water or food to reduce the desire to procreate so that eventually the population of the enemy country would be reduced in a deliberate zero growth population control. Conversely, LRH or its analogues could be employed to create havoc, with citizens' minds fixed on procreation and nothing else. There is a treasure trove of plots for thriller writers in the possibilities being opened up by this new aphrodisiac from the brain.

To most people, of course, LRH is of far more immediate interest on a personal level. "I think there are an awful lot of people who have problems sexually and I think if their sexual problems are overcome a lot of their personal problems would be overcome," says Robert L. Moss, a University of Texas physiologist pioneering in LRH research.

It is no secret, furthermore, that sexual interest declines with age, with a disparity between men and women of the same age. Says Dr. Moss: "The number of forty- to fifty-year-old men who have a decrease in sexual function while their wives are sexually active is probably high. Also, men in stressful situations, such as sales positions, have decreased sex lives. Our aim is to help restore sexual function."

A highly promising beginning has already been made. At the University of Texas health sciences center in Dallas, LRH has been administered to married men twenty-five to forty years of age whose sexual activity had been blocked by psychological causes. Results have been highly encouraging, with sexual activity returning. In ongoing studies the hormone is already being given by mouth and as a nasal spray.

In tests at Saint Bartholomew Hospital in London, LRH restored sexual potency, fertility, and spermatogenesis in a number of impotent males. When LRH was injected into young men fourteen to twenty-two years old in whom puberty was delayed because of brain tumors, complete sexual functioning appeared in four to five weeks. In older, previously impotent males, LRH therapy for a year or less produced potency and elevated sperm counts from zero to 500 million. Even more dramatically, an Asian exile from Uganda who had been rendered impotent after his pituitary gland had been irradiated to correct a form of gigantism known as acromegaly succeeded in impregnating his wife after sixty-four weeks of LRH therapy. The result was a healthy baby boy with no evidence of congenital malformations.

This aphrodisiac from the brain is so new that it has not been deliberately tested yet on frigid women. There is no doubt, though, that it works in women. The application of LRH as a spectacular new sex pill came about, in fact, through the hormone's initial use to induce ovulation in previously infertile women.

Such women have in the past been treated with "fertility drugs," substances that mimic the effects of the pituitary hormones on the ovary. The problem with such treatments is the difficulty of controlling doses so that only one egg is released from the ovary at a time. The result has often been the near-tragedy of multiple births with very few, if any, of the babies surviving. In contrast, LRH triggers the body's own ovulation mechanism, liberating one egg at a time. In fact, this has been successfully accomplished in several previously infertile women in both the United States and Europe. These women have already given birth as a result of the LRH treatment.

On the other hand, antagonists of LRH block ovulation. In long-acting form (yet to be developed), they would have to be taken only once a month—a nearly perfect birth-control pill.

Scientists knew that LRH is produced in the hypothalamus, one of the brain's major control centers, and that it acts on the adjoining pituitary lodged in the base of the brain to promote formation in the pituitary of the two reproductive hormones, luteinizing hormone (LH) and follicle-stimulating hormone (FSH).

A surge of these hormones triggers ovulation and stimulates the ovaries to produce estrogen and progesterone, the most widely known female sex hormones. What the scientists didn't know was that LRH stimulated sexual behavior as well as ovulation, revealing a fascinating link between brain, behavior, and body. When they found that sexual activity of women given LRH as an ovulating agent was enhanced, they quickly began investigating LRH's role as an aphrodisiac.

Experiments at first were conducted with female rats. It was clearly shown by Moss and other scientists that LRH stimulated the animals' sexual behavior. The scientists then traced the specific pathways followed by LRH in its action on the brain. They found that the hormone not only diffuses from the hypothalamus to the pituitary but also that some of the substance also goes directly to the areas of the brain associated with sexual arousal and mating. If proof was ever needed of the old folk saying that sex is a chemical reaction, Moss and his associates produced it when they tracked LRH molecules to the pleasure center in the ancient part of the brain that controls sexual arousal.

Studying the binding of LRH by neurons in the brains of different animal species—fish, amphibians, birds, rats, rhesus monkeys—researchers found remarkable similarities in where the hormone binds despite the species differences. The hormone unerringly seeks out certain structures in the phylogenetically ancient part of the forebrain, in the hypothalamus, and in certain other brain regions. Scientists concluded that sex hormone receptors exist in all the vertebrates.

Pinpointing such pleasure centers, or specific networks of neurons that control basic emotions and drives (sex, hunger, thirst, sleep, arousal, attention, social play, and predatory attack) ranks among the great recent achievements of neurobiology. All these needs, moods, or emotions can be called forth or suppressed. Perhaps the most dramatic public demonstration of the effect was when José Delgado stopped an enraged bull dead in its tracks with a signal transmitted by radio to a receiver attached to electrodes implanted in the bull's head. (Delgado was then at Yale but now continues his work in Spain.)

Where sexual behavior is concerned, scientists found that a rat—or a man, for that matter—will endlessly stimulate his pleasure centers in the brain by pushing a lever that produces the signal—forgetting the need to eat and sleep. Scientists have put this new knowledge to work. In one case, a young man who wanted to reverse his homosexuality did so through electrical stimulation of his arousal center and simultaneously viewing a display of slides of attractive young women.

Not many people would want electrodes inserted in their heads even for constant enjoyment of sexual satisfaction more intense than the real thing. But now we have LRH. It performs the same task as electrical stimulation, though whereas electrical stimulation works instantaneously, chemical stimulation by LRH takes about a half-hour to an hour to work. And the new sex pill can simply be taken by mouth or as a nasal spray.

LRH is the most spectacular new mood-made-to-order drug to come from the brain, but it isn't the only one. In fact, the brain is turning out to be a treasure trove of these fantasy-tinged mood and mind medications. In addition to LRH, the brain produces a great variety of chemical messengers whose discovery and application hold profound implications not only for people suffering from behavioral disorders—sexual dysfunction, senility, hyperkineticism, schizophrenia—but for normal people as well. The newly found code words of behavior control a whole range of emotions and abilities, from enhancement of visual attention to induction of sleep. These brain chemicals are all peptides, or small protein molecules. In effect, they are fractions of hormones that act directly on the brain, just as LRH does. Also like LRH, they apparently accomplish their activation task by diffusing through networks of specific neurons (those centers of behavior control) to convey long-lasting messages that modify and modulate behavior.

These chemical code words of behavior appear to be engaged in a different and broader form of communication than are the neurotransmitters. The better-known neurotransmitters, such as noradrenaline, serotonin, and dopamine, are small molecules that travel exceedingly short distances to cause rapid, momentary changes in the excitability of a neuron. The peptides, on the other hand, act as hormones in the brain, carrying executive commands to groups of nerve cells by diffusing their more complicated molecules across longer distances and causing longer-lasting changes in the excitability of specific nerve cells. The current view is that control of such complex states as moods by a single neurotransmitter is unlikely.

It's all the more remarkable that these chemical code words of behavior occur in amounts so minute that, to get a few milligrams of a pure releasing factor that acts on the pituitary to release into the bloodstream a hormone that stimulates the thyroid, scientists had to extract the material from the hypothalami of about 1.5 *million* sheep and pigs. Nature does not waste its code words where behavioral control is concerned.

The idea that hormones can affect the way we feel or how we act has been around for some time. The depression or irritability many women feel just before or during menstruation, for instance, or at menopause correlates with the times when estrogen levels are low. It has long been obvious, too, that the brain can influence the hormones of the body. An emotional disturbance can make a woman miss a menstrual period. Women can also undergo false pregnancies. In animals, more bizarre phenomena can occur. Pregnant female mice will, for instance, abort if a strange male comes near.

How the brain was directly involved in influencing moods and behavior wasn't known, however. It was long thought that the body's master gland was the pituitary, the pea-sized organ tucked away in a bony socket just beneath the hypothalamus and joined to this full-fledged part of the brain by a scrawny stalk. The front lobe of the pituitary secretes a large number of hormones that act on the target organs in the body. These include the adrenal glands, the thyroid, the breasts, and of course the sex glands—the ovaries in women and testes in men. Another hormone from the pituitary, the growth hormone, has a generalized effect on the body.

Because the pituitary is housed so close to the brain and in particular to the hypothalamus, the notion that the brain influences the pituitary via the hypothalamus has been around for many years. The puzzle was how the two communicated. The nervous connections between the hypothalamus and the pituitary are sparse.

Geoffrey Harris of Oxford University finally found a pathway. Harris suspected that the rich supply of blood vessels between the hypothalamus and the pituitary might serve as a conduit for chemical factors that could control the release of the various hormones of the anterior pituitary. It was a brilliant intuition, and Harris proved his point by interrupting the blood flow to the pituitary in laboratory animals and by transplanting the pituitary to other sites in the body. Only when fed with blood fresh from the hypothalamus would the gland release its hormones.

The brain's master gland, it became clear, was not the pituitary but the hypothalamus, an unusual organ because of the extraordinary array of inputs it receives from all over the nervous system and the brain and because of the wide range of bodily functions over which it holds sway. These include temperature regulation, water balance, sleep, and various emotional reactions as well as sex, growth, lactation, and stress. The hypothalamus controls the latter functions by neurohormones.

Once the notion of the command substances known as chemical releasing factors became accepted, a race began to isolate and identify them. And what a race it turned out to be, involving in one laboratory alone the use of 5 million fragments of sheep brains weighing a total of more than 500 tons. A keen sense of rivalry seldom equaled even in the competitive world of scientific research developed between the two principal researchers and laboratories that were the front runners in the race, Roger Guillemin, now at the Salk Institute in La Jolla, California, and Andrew Schally, now at Tulane University Medical School in New Orleans. In the end they divided the honors fairly evenly, sharing the 1977 Nobel Prize in physiology and medicine for their remarkable achievements.

Guillemin scored the first success, isolating minute quantities of the releasing factor that regulates the secretion by the pituitary of the hormone that stimulates the thyroid. This is the hormone that in man prompts the thyroid gland to release its two major hormones, thyroxin and triiodothyronie. Both of these have generalized effects on growth, development, and metabolism. This first releasing factor, identified in 1969, was called TRF. Two years later, first Schally and then shortly afterward Guillemin identified LRH.

The availability of LRH and of very sensitive assay systems for it in the body have made possible in the last year or so an entirely new understanding of the intricate interplay of hormones that constitute the reproductive cycle in women. It turns out that there is both negative and positive feedback from the ovary to the pituitary. This feedback is mediated by the two sex hormones estrogen and progesterone, supplied by the ovary to the pituitary and hypothalamus during the woman's monthly cycle. Their effects are exerted both by altering the output of LRH from the hypothalamus and by changing the sensitivity of the pituitary to the LRH.

The involvement of the hypothalamus, part of the brain, in these feedback loops explains how the mind can interfere in the normal workings of the monthly cycle. For instance, a woman who exhibits a false pregnancy sends out from the hypothalamus larger amounts of LRH than normal. On the other hand, when a woman skips her normal menstrual period because of some unusual event in her life, it is because the output of LRH is lower than normal.

It is fitting that the word *hormone* comes from a Greek word meaning "to rouse to activity." Women who lack sexual desire do not produce enough LRH to diffuse to those centers of sexual arousal in the brain. Women who never ovulate and are as a result infertile may be that way because of a near-total failure of the hypothalamus to send its LRH signal down the pituitary stalk.

As so often happens in science, it was a roundabout route that led researchers to realize that hormones can act directly on the brain. The idea that they could do so was revolutionary, for scientists had thought that hormones influenced only the target glands. From this mistaken notion arose all kinds of myths, such as the belief that the timing of the menopause was controlled by depletion of egg cells in the ovary—a kind of drying up of hormones. We now know that like other key events in life this female change of life is controlled by the brain (see Chapter 7). It is also clear now that, in a very real sense, glands are an extension of the brain because they are controlled by it and hormones made in the brain diffuse through the brain to influence moods and behavior.

The story of how that knowledge was discovered began about fifteen years ago when a young Harvard-educated research physician, Abba J. Kastin, became intrigued by the enigmatic role in human biology of a hormone that controls pigmentation in frogs and other amphibians. It is called MSH, for melanocyte-stimulating hormone, melanocytes being the pigment-producing cells. In amphibians MSH has obvious adaptive value in facilitating camouflage through a rapid pigmentary change. Sudden changes in the environment, such as the presence of a predator, often signal danger, and an amphibian's ability to detect the change and camouflage itself is vital to its survival.

But what was MSH doing in man? No racial differences in MSH levels between Negroes and Caucasians had been observed, which suggested that a skin-coloring function in man was unlikely. Kastin reasoned that in man MSH must have an adaptive function of a different type acting directly on the brain. He found that the brain had evolved elaborate mechanisms for controlled release of the hormone, and it seemed unlikely that nature would have gone to all that trouble for a substance that had no function in the body. Kastin also discovered that the human body contained about as much MSH as is present in the body of the frog.

While doing research in Sweden in 1966, Kastin found that half the women in a test group given small doses of MSH showed changes in their brain waves as recorded by an encephalograph. This was an exciting lead that MSH acted directly on the brain. Following up this interesting discovery, Kastin, with his collaborators Curt Sandman and Lyle Miller, showed in 1971 that small doses of MSH improve visual attention and retention in healthy human volunteers. In later tests they found that MSH also reduces anxiety. In 1976 Kastin and his colleagues showed that MSH helped the mentally retarded solve problems, such as remembering and then drawing geometric shapes, in about half the time it would have normally taken them. In mental retardation, as well as in schizophrenia and other types of mental illness, inability to concentrate on the task at hand is what hinders learning. Not surprisingly, Kastin feels that giving MSH to people with those conditions would be beneficial. The results obtained with MSH were far better and more specific than the much more generalized stimulation that can be obtained with amphetamine pep pills.

By acting on the visual area of the brain, the hormone improves the brain's information-processing ability. MSH appears to act by activating an enzyme that makes the membrane more porous and by synthesizing protein—metabolic effects that, in turn, energize the nerve cell into greater activity. Measuring the effects of the hormone fragment on brain activity in people, investigators found that the frequency of their theta waves, associated with a state of arousal and alertness, can be increased by administering tiny amounts of the hormone. MSH thus speeds transmission of signals in the brain, boosting the state of arousal. That in turn enhances the motivation produced by specific visual cues and leads to improved performance.

At about the same time that Kastin was doing his early research on MSH, a group of Dutch researchers led by pharmacologist David de Wied made a puzzling discovery about another hormone, ACTH (adrenocorticotropic hormone). While trying to trace how the release of ACTH is inhibited by the pituitary, they found that secretion of the hormone was reduced in some stress situations but not in others. Stress with high emotional content, such as exposure to a strange environment, reduced the release of ACTH, whereas its levels remained normal in systemic stress such as is produced by an injury.

Following up, the scientists tested rats for both learning ability and memory retention and found that administration of ACTH helped the animals remember tasks they had learned. The researchers also found that the animals' ability to learn, impaired by partial removal of the pituitary, could be restored by giving the animals ACTH.

Since ACTH was known to act on the adrenal glands, the researchers at first assumed that these glands mediated the learning effect. But removal of the adrenals did not impair learning. The conclusion that ACTH acted directly on the brain seemed inescapable.

To be certain, the scientists tried MSH, which is similar in structure to ACTH but does not affect the adrenals. With the pituitaries of the rats totally removed, MSH had the same restorative effect on learning as ACTH. This finding supported Kastin's early notion that MSH acted directly on the brain.

The researchers found that only a tiny fraction of the total MSH or ACTH molecule directly affects behavior. ACTH, as one scientist said, is "a rather flexible molecule with its amino acid 'letters' arranged into a 'sentence' that is subdivided into 'words' with different biological meanings." Only one of these "words," merely six amino acids long, directly affects behavior. Exactly the same sequence occurs in the MSH molecule.

De Wied introduced the term *neuropeptide* for these mood-control segments, to distinguish them from the conventional components of the whole hormone molecule that act on target organs outside the brain to produce more diffuse physiological effects. "Neuropeptides are involved in acquisition and maintenance of new behavioral patterns," de Wied says. "They facilitate registration, consolidation, repression, and retrieval of information, which makes possible the selection of adequate behavior." He thinks that many neuropeptides act upon the old emotional brain, with all its complex and interacting influences on personality, motivation, and fear. The discovery of neuropeptides clearly has explosive implications for controlling the behavior of not only the sick but of healthy people as well.

Working closely with scientists from the Dutch drug firm Organon, the de Wied group at the University of Utrecht has also delineated the remarkable activities of neuropeptide fractions of the hormones vasopressin and oxytocin. These two hormones, like many others, are synthesized in the hypothalamus and then stored in the pituitary until needed.

Outside the brain, vasopressin regulates water metabolism and blood pressure, and oxytocin facilitates childbirth and lactation. But in the brain, the direct effects of the neuropeptide fractions of these hormones are dramatically different. The behavioral components of vasopressin have a long-term "cementing" effect on consolidation of information. The oxytocin fragment has an opposite effect, repressing and erasing information, just like those science-fictional drugs Stanislaw Lem wrote about. De Wied says that with oxytocin we may finally have a means of treating people with the concentration-camp syndrome, the inability to forget gruesome experiences.

De Wied's team has synthesized an analogue, or chemical copy, of the behavioral portion of the ACTH molecule that is a thousand times more powerful than the natural neuropeptide. Now being manufactured by Organon for experimental use, the analogue can be taken by mouth. De Wied feels that ACTH and vasopressin may be useful as correctives—to improve learning abilities of hyperkinetic children, for instance, and to boost motivation and failing memories of the elderly. Encouraged by finding that an ACTH analogue improved learning in old rats, the Dutch scientists are now testing the neuropeptides on senile people.

Kastin and the other members of the scientific "peptide generation" are understandably elated by these developments. Kastin works in a one-story cement-block animal building at the Veterans Administration Hospital next to the Tulane University Medical School in New Orleans. He is associated with both institutions. The anteroom to his office is filled with cages full of frogs, and toy frogs, gifts from associates, adorn his cramped office. Kastin flatly declares, "The age of the hypothalamic peptide has arrived."

Indeed, more and more neuropeptides are being discovered. One of the most spectacular recent finds has been the endorphins, the brain's own opiatelike pain-killers.

Whereas the presence of chemical neurotransmitters that convey messages between neurons in the brain was originally inferred through their activity in the peripheral nervous system, the endorphins were discovered in a more planned approach that offers much promise for the future of mood control.

The presence of endorphins was suggested by a number of scientists who speculated that the brain must make its own morphinelike pain-killer. Otherwise, they wondered, why should morphine, a plant substance that would not normally find its way into the brain, act on the brain? Morphine apparently acted by binding to receptors on the surface of brain cells, the way most medications act. It was unlikely, the scientists reasoned, that receptors would have evolved in the brain just to suit a plant substance. They figured that the brain made its own pain-killer similar in structure to morphine.

Possibly, such a natural pain-killer filled an evolutionary need—a wounded caveman could escape from enemies without being disabled by suffering. The existence of such a substance would also explain the brief, and sometimes not so brief, painfree period commonly experienced by wounded soldiers, injured sportsmen, and other people in stressful situations.

On the surface, the effects of stress, fear, and arousal on pain perception look paradoxical. Moderate anxiety increases the response to pain, whereas high levels of anxiety, including terror or fear, *decrease* the response to pain. But in terms of survival such a response makes a great deal of sense. Perception of pain depends on environmental situations and on the state of arousal at a particular moment. As one scientist explains it, "Thus, being hit in the mouth by a mugger, in a perhaps life-or-death situation, may cause little or no immediate pain, while the slightest touch by a dentist of a patient's tooth may readily elicit wincing."

It is now clear that high stress and anxiety trigger a release of endorphins with an analgesic response to painful stimuli. Acupuncture anesthesia apparently works through endorphins, too, explaining at last a long-standing mystery. The needles prompt the brain to release endorphins, which then block the pathways of pain.

The discovery of the body's own pain-killers could also call for some changes in the way we label people. Is a man brave because he produces a large supply of endorphins that make him insensitive to pain? Is he a coward because of an endorphin deficiency?

Not until 1973 did Solomon Snyder and his associates at Johns Hopkins pinpoint the location of opiate receptors in the brain. Not surprisingly, they found them concentrated in parts of the brain associated with the pathways of pain. Snyder and his colleagues showed in laboratory experiments that when they introduced ground calves' brains into a solution containing morphine receptors, the material would bind to the morphine receptors, competing with exogenous morphine, which was also in solution. It became clear that there existed a substance in the calves' brains similar to morphine.

At this point, the search took one of those odd turns that make science an adventure. In 1964, Choh Hao Li, a pioneer in hormone research at the University of California's San Francisco Medical Center, discovered a new hormone. It consisted of ninety-one amino acids and seemed to mobilize fat, or lipids, in the body, so Li accordingly called it lipotropin.

Searching for a more specific function for the substance, Li decided to look for it in the camel. Since the camel is a very skinny animal, Li guessed he might get some interesting insights into how lipotropin worked. Li happened to have an Iraqi scientist working in the lab whom he asked to bring back some dried camel pituitaries from his next trip home. The man returned—with five hundred of them—and, presumably, a convincing story for the customs inspector.

Li and his colleagues found no complete lipotropin in the camel material. But they did find that the camel degrades lipotropin to MSH, the anxiety and stress-reducing hormone that Kastin and de Wied have worked with. In the course of their work, Li and his associates also found a fragment of the lipotropin molecule in the camel, a shorter peptide of thirty-one amino acids that was structurally identical to the last one-third of the lipotropin molecule. The function of this substance remained a mystery until December 18, 1975, when British scientist John J. Hughes and his associates reported in the journal *Nature* that they had discovered an even smaller peptide with morphinelike properties in the brain of the pig. They called it enkephalin ("from the brain," in Greek).

To Li and his colleagues, enkephalin looked like a word straight from the chemical sentence they had fished out of those Iraqi camels, for Hughes's enkephalin was chemically identical to a small segment of the camel material. Now enlightened about the nature of his find, Li named his camel material *beta-endorphin,* for endogenous morphine. He has since shown that it has about thirty times the potency of morphine when injected directly into the brains of mice and rats. The high concentration of beta-endorphins in the camel's brain explains, he says, why the camel is such a hardy animal. "You can kick it," marvels Li, "even stick a knife in its side, and it won't feel the pain."

Few biological substances have generated as much feverish activity as the brain's own opiates. Scientists are churning out papers in the journals as they keep learning more and more about the manifold activities of the endorphins, which appear to mediate a large number of brain functions. "Our excitement about this molecule lies in the fact that we may have uncovered a whole new vocabulary of chemical signals," says Floyd Bloom, a biochemist at the Salk Institute. "Nothing has excited neuroscientists as much for a long time."

The biggest surprise about the endorphins is that they may hold the key to schizophrenia and other mental illnesses (see Chapter 4, Psychopharmacology: Fighting Depression). "What we observe with beta-endorphins," says Bloom, "suggests that if the human pituitary excreted these substances in slightly higher than normal amounts, you'd have something very much like catatonic schizophrenia." In humans, endorphins occur in such minute quantities that they are hard to detect. But some scientists think they have located endorphinlike material in the spinal fluid of schizophrenics.

Pursuing that lead, researchers have begun to treat schizophrenics with antiopiate compounds. One Swedish scientist, Lars Terenius of the University of Uppsala, recently treated six patients, four of whom had auditory hallucinations. All four stopped hearing voices within minutes of treatment.

So many and varied are the actions of these brain hormones that there is even a suspicion that endorphins turn sleep on and off, for within the large precursor lipotropin molecule discovered by Li there are not only activators but also antagonists of all sorts of physiological activities. A fragment called gamma endorphin, for instance, makes animals irritable and hypersensitive, whereas the alpha portion has a most soothing effect. There are obvious possibilities for mood-control drugs here.

Floyd Bloom has shown the remarkable action of beta-endorphin. Given to rats, it made them stiff as boards. So rigid were the animals that they remained fixed in position, with tails outstretched horizontally, even when placed on edges of metal bookends. Hanging stiffly in the air as if frozen, the animals supported themselves only at the neck and the base of the tail. Beta-endorphin is the same substance that camels manufacture in large quantities by breaking down the lipotropin molecule, to protect themselves against their drivers' kicks and other rough treatment and stresses they are exposed to.

Neither camels nor men, however, become addicted to their own morphinelike pain-killers, because the endorphins, like most body substances but unlike synthetic morphine, are rapidly degraded.

A nonaddictive pain-killer is only one of a cornucopia of new drugs that will come out of endorphin research. The discovery that a substance manufactured in the body has powerful pain-killing ability and other opiate properties without morphine's undesirable side effects and habit-forming qualities has far-reaching implications not only for the relief of pain but also for a deeper understanding of narcotics addiction and mental disorders. In addicts, endorphins could relieve the symptoms of morphine withdrawal. In normal people, endorphinlike drugs could induce euphoria and reduce anxiety as opiates do, but without their side effects. All kinds of nonaddictive euphoriants based on endorphins will be synthesized; the race is already on among drug companies.

"With our knowledge about the receptor-opiate interaction," says Solomon Snyder, the pioneer in opiate-receptor research from Johns Hopkins, "we can rapidly screen new drugs simply in a test tube, with drug and receptor added together. We will know right off if the drugs act on the receptors or not. This enormously improves the chances for rapid development of new drugs along this line."

One scientist, Irving Johnson, a physician and vice president of the Eli Lilly research laboratories, explains why the lipotropin molecule is so rich in content. "Nature is rather like a plumber," says Dr. Johnson, "who takes all his tools along with him on a job and then uses a few specific ones when he gets there." Out of this plumber's tool box, scientists plan to extract a whole range of new drugs, including nonaddictive pain-killers that could also be used to wean addicts away from dangerous narcotics.

As if to illustrate further the versatility of the messengers from the brain, more and more neuropeptides are being uncovered. Angiotensin produces thirst so strong that after an injection an animal stops whatever it is doing, proceeds to a water spout, and starts drinking. A starving animal that has only just been allowed to eat stops eating to look for water. A laboratory rat given the hormone overcomes its natural fear of man and struggles to reach the water spout, even when manually restrained.

From the brains of sleeping cats, collaborating American and Mexican researchers have recently extracted two peptides that are present only during the dreaming phase of sleep and not when the animals are awake. (The chemicals are extracted from the brains of sleeping cats through minute, surgically implanted tubes connected to a small pump.) By injecting these substances into the brains of cats that were awake, scientists have induced the more rapid and more frequent appearance of dream-filled periods in the animals. These dream periods are measured with instruments that detect the so-called rapid eye movement, or REM, sleep.

This most important phase of sleep is severely altered in many psychiatric patients and obliterated by all current sleeping pills. Scientists think that a natural brain chemical responsible for dreaming sleep will soon be isolated in the human brain. It could then be synthesized to produce sleeping pills to remedy insomnia without interfering with dreaming.

Similarly, from the brains of goats deprived of sleep, Harvard scientists have extracted a substance that increases the duration of sleep in rats. It, too, appears to be a peptide, as does a similar substance obtained by Japanese scientists from the brains of one thousand rats.

Perhaps the strangest of all neuropeptides so far discovered is scotophobin (after the Greek for "fear of the dark"). Georges Ungar, now at the University of Tennessee Medical Center in Memphis, and his colleagues trained four thousand rats to fear the dark and then tested different fractions of material extracted from their brains on untrained rats. They narrowed down the extract to an eleven-amino-acid molecule that imparts the fear of the dark for a whole week after a single injection. Scotophobin comes close to substances in Stanislaw Lem's fictional society, where "books are no longer read but eaten, not made of paper but of some informational substance; fully digestible, sugar-coated."

Scotophobin could be used to bring nocturnal animals into the open. For example, in rat-infested areas, where rats have become resistant to poison, scotophobin could be mixed with food left out for the rats; the neuropeptide would make the rats appear in daylight so that they could be killed by other means. And scotophobin slipped into enemy soldiers' food or drink would make them reluctant to fight after dark.

Possibly because of its science-fiction flavor, scotophobin's discovery in 1970 was greeted with skepticism. But the recent finding that the brain appears to be packed with neuropeptides acting as behavior codes places scotophobin on a solid scientific footing. Besides, its activity has been confirmed in many laboratories in interesting ways. Not only do untrained mice and rats given scotophobin suddenly acquire a fear of the dark, but in an experiment in Belgium a fish that normally lives in the dark under rocks now spends its time in the light near the surface.

More recently, Ungar has discovered a number of other learning-induced peptides. Among them are ameletin (Greek for "indifferent"), which induces habituation to a sound stimulus in rats; antendorphin, which produces a tolerance to morphine; and two chromodiopsins, extracted from the brains of ten thousand goldfish trained to avoid the colors green and blue, respectively.

Ungar is trying to break the peptides' chemical behavior code, a task he considers more prodigious than the deciphering of the genetic alphabet. "The genetic code has four amino acid 'letters,' but here we have twenty," says Ungar. "We probably have an innate vocabulary for a certain number of instinctive behaviors—certain peptides are probably formed at birth. The others probably are formed from these innate words and combined into sentences. Scotophobin, for instance, may be put together from three or four shorter peptides."

Despite the difficulties of breaking down the code, some tantalizing clues are emerging. Ungar's two-color-discrimination peptides, for instance, both consist of thirteen amino acids. A sequence of nine units is the same in both peptides and apparently tells the fish to avoid electric shock which they receive if they don't choose the right-colored pathway, whereas the other four amino acids represent, respectively, the colors blue and green. The reward of deciphering these and other code words would be the resolution of such intriguing questions as what constitutes, for instance, a command to remember or one to forget.

If Ungar is right in his belief that millions of different behavioral peptides can be formed in the brain, there will be enough work for generations of brain researchers. The specificity of the brain peptides discovered so far seems to support Ungar's view. Ameletin, for instance, is produced only in response to a ringing electric bell but not the sound of a gong. (That sound apparently produces another, yet-to-be-discovered peptide.) Another group of scientists has extracted a brain peptide from rats that had been trained by means of electric shock to remain on a platform rather than step down, illustrating an apparently unlimited specificity of the brain peptides.

The brain peptides hold great promise as mind drugs not only because of their remarkably specific and practically unlimited information content but also because, being the brain's own "drugs," they are essentially nontoxic. For instance, the fraction of vasopressin that has a marked effect on behavior doesn't act on the kidneys or on the cardiovascular system, as the complete vasopressin molecule does. Similarly, LRH analogues in doses one thousand times greater than those required to get pituitary effects show no side effects. Another advantage is the neuropeptides' relatively simple structure—most of them have already been synthesized. Before we know it, that nasal spray to arouse sexual desire may become one of the hottest and most sought-after black-market drugs.

It is important to remember, of course, that environmental influences, a person's experiences and moods, can in turn trigger hormone secretion and its accompanying behavior. A person who is nervous or anxious secretes ACTH, for instance, which influences the adrenal steroids. Even a sound can set off a flow of hormones. Control of lactation, for example, is directly conditioned to milk letdown on hearing an infant cry, and not just on the actual physical stimulation of sucking. Even the gonadotropins that regulate sex hormone secretion have been shown to be influenced by an animal's behavioral state.

The word *castrate,* in the sense of a violent confrontation between two people, is also apparently literally true, because it can have the functional effect for a period of time of reducing the flow of sex hormones and functionally castrating the person. A male monkey decisively defeated by a dominant male, for instance, will experience a temporary shutdown of the gonadotropin secretion. But give him a compatible female companion and he'll recover much more rapidly than he would otherwise.

Bruce McEwen, a researcher at Rockefeller University, says, "Once it is understood that behavior influences hormone secretion, that normal secretion not only influences bodily function but also brain function, then a basis emerges for understanding a lot of the psychosomatic illnesses."

Or put another way, if the old folk saying "It's all in your head" means that there is nothing to it, the story of neuropeptides demonstrates dramatically that there is almost everything to what *is* in your mind.

CHAPTER THREE

Food and Your Mood

"Eat and you'll feel better."

—The mother of Dr. Arnold J. Mandell, cochairman of the department of psychiatry, the University of California at San Diego, instructing him when he was a small boy

In some ways, modern science is just beginning to discover what folk wisdom arrived at ages ago. Laymen have known or suspected that food influences our moods—most parents know, for instance, that when a child misses a meal, that child will often become irritable and impolite. Grown-ups are affected, too, and will say and do things when hungry and irritated that they wouldn't think of doing two minutes after eating.

Now science is coming in on the coattails of this folk wisdom. In recent work that relates to brain chemistry, for instance, scientists have begun to show that what we eat may have a lot to do with how we act. Neurotransmitters and neuropeptides, the brain's chemical signal carriers, are synthesized from building blocks in the food we consume. Tryptophan, for instance, is an amino acid precursor of serotonin, the reptilian brain's favorite repressive neurotransmitter. Rats fed a diet of corn, which is deficient in tryptophan, become hypersensitive to pain and extremely aggressive. Rats that never killed mice before suddenly turn into killers when their brain serotonin becomes depleted.

The connection between food and mood has always seemed highly logical to many people, but until just recently conventional science denied that such a connection existed. In fact, some ultraconservative psychiatrists still deny it exists. Until some recent experiments began to disprove the idea, it was widely believed by scientists that the brain lived in splendid isolation from the rest of the body and that the body, in fact, protected the brain from malnutrition at the expense of less important organs.

Since that was the prevailing belief, scientists didn't bother to experiment to disprove the idea, which may strike laymen as a curious way of approaching science. Is science supposed to be bold exploration of the unknown, or is dogged defense of entrenched views its more regular mode of operation? Unfortunately, more often than not it's the latter. And medicine has been especially guilty of scoffing at anything new.

"The prevailing view when I went to medical school and in many places still today," says Dr. Richard J. Wurtman of the department of nutrition at the Massachusetts Institute of Technology (MIT), "was that the brain was so important that it was isolated from the rest of the body. You had to use a sledgehammer if you wanted to do anything to the brain. But now we recognize that not only is the brain amenable to component changes in the blood level, but that it actually passively reflects those changes which, in turn, depend on the diet. Everyone expected malnutrition to affect the brain. What wasn't expected was that *normal* nutrition could affect it."

Now scientists at MIT and elsewhere are trying to figure out what foods would be best for the brain to control moods. They can already offer some suggestions. Manic-depressives, for instance, may have to alter their diets with their moods. When feeling depressed, they might do well to stay away from eggs, soybeans, and liver, because they all contain choline, a building block of the neurotransmitter acetylcholine. On the other hand, such foods may suppress their episodes of mania (see Chapter 4, Fighting Depression).

Laymen have also anticipated scientists in the practical application of such knowledge. For instance, people who drink milk before bedtime seem to be on the right track, since milk contains sleep-inducing tryptophan. And Charles Dickens displayed a remarkable insight into diet and brain chemistry. When Scrooge sees the ghost of Marley in *A Christmas Carol,* the ghost asks him, "Why do you doubt your senses?" Scrooge answers: "Because a little thing affects them. A slight disorder of the stomach makes them cheats. You may be an undigested bit of beef, a blot of mustard, a crumb of cheese, a fragment of an underdone potato. There's more gravy than grave about you, whatever you are!"

Some people do get vivid dreams after eating cheese—raising some interesting questions about the connection between tyramine in cheese and ergot, the rye fungus from which LSD is made.

The expression "feeling one's oats" may also have something to do with brain chemistry. It may have originated with horsemen who observed long ago that eating oats makes horses frisky. Samuel Johnson, writing on his travels in Scotland, reported commenting disdainfully to Scotsmen whom he saw eating oats: "In England, we give oats to horses." He got an appropriate rejoinder: "Yes, Dr. Johnson, that's why you have such fine horses in England and we have such fine men in Scotland!"

Like the rest of the body, the brain derives its nutrients from food. All told, more than forty different vitamins, trace elements, minerals, amino acids, and other food components go into operating the chemical factories that are our cells. The brain is even more of a chemical factory than most other organs—it is an electric computer submerged in a chemical cauldron, 90 percent of which is water. Hence, any imbalance in natural nutrients or the presence of poisonous foreign substances can affect the brain in startling ways. The offending substances have for some especially sensitive people only to be present in minute amounts.

For instance, Dr. Ben F. Feingold, who pioneered much of the research into the impact of food additives on hyperkinetic children, tells of a boy whose aggressive attacks were set off by eating a single hot dog. Minute amounts of additives in the hot dog precipitated the outbursts, which stopped after the boy was put on an additivefree diet.

A highly unbalanced diet can lead to a loss of memory. When investigators deprived a group of patients of the amino acids phenylalanine and tyrosine to starve rapidly growing tumors, the patients developed an acute disturbance of memory. To some extent this memory loss resembled the so-called Scoville-Milner syndrome, which is characterized by bilateral destruction of the medial temporal lobes. The patients also showed considerable confusion, displaying delusions characteristic of delirium. But when a full amino acid diet was supplied again, the patients regained their memories.

Similarly, chronic alcoholics who replace food with drink suffer damage to memory. This is true of alcoholics who begin to substitute alcohol for food to the point where they deprive themselves of the B vitamins, particularly vitamin B_1, or thiamine. Unless thiamine is administered early enough, the disturbance proceeds to loss of past memories and an inability to form new memories or learn new things.

Once the amnesic syndrome develops, however, it's difficult to counteract. Indicating the almost permanent nature of the brain damage, at this late stage thiamine restores only about 20 percent of the memory loss. Putting these patients on a high carbohydrate diet or giving them glucose without treating the vitamin deficiency first can make matters worse because the need for thiamine is further increased.*

Many other severe effects can be produced by vitamin deficiencies. Scurvy occurs with lack of vitamin C, which the human body does not make but must obtain from food sources. Pellagra, often accompanied by insanity, is miraculously cured by niacinamide (vitamin B_3) and other vitamins. Early in this century, pellagra raged among the poor in the southern states, people whose diets consisted mainly of corn.

Deficiencies in trace elements such as zinc can lead to mental illness. On the other hand, too much mercury in the brain can lead to suicide. Suicides are particularly high among dentists, who use mercury in their work.

Vitamins, minerals, and trace elements perform highly specific jobs in metabolism. No fewer than fifty-one metals, from aluminum to zirconium, are now known to be present in the body in varying amounts. Without them, in trace amounts, no plant or animal, including man, could live. Iron, magnesium, calcium, chromium, cobalt, copper, and zinc are known to be essential to life, and vanadium, nickel,

*There is a good scientific reason why a thiamine deficiency affects memory. In animal tissues, thiamine assumes the form of thiamine diphosphate (TDP), which accounts for 80 percent of the vitamin. Thiamine makes up the rest. TDP acts as a well-known coenzyme, or helper, in the synthesis of RNA, which in turn is now known to be involved in memory formation (see Chapter 6 on memory).

and tin are thought to be. Often incorporated into proteins, metals serve as catalysts that initiate or assist in biological reactions. Each of the four iron atoms in a hemoglobin molecule, for instance, is a "handle" to which oxygen molecules become attached, to be carried throughout the body in the red pigment of the blood.

Over the millennia, organisms developed delicate balancing, or homeostatic, mechanisms to regulate the rate at which essential trace metals are incorporated into their tissues. But in general, organisms, including man, failed to develop comparable defenses against the heavier metals that perform no beneficial biological function. These metals are toxic in their elemental forms, especially if they are absorbed as small particles, and become even more hazardous in organic compounds, which are more rapidly absorbed into the body and tend to concentrate in nerve tissue. A notable example is methyl mercury, which is far more dangerous than mercury in its familiar metallic form. Another is tetraethyl lead, which, being readily soluble in fats, is particularly damaging to nerve centers and to the brain. Both these substances can be unknowingly absorbed in contaminated food or from polluted air.

Vitamins, for their part, are crucially important to metabolism because they often serve as coenzymes. Enzymes are proteins that act as catalysts of biochemical reactions, and coenzymes are the helpers in this process. Today, ten vitamins are known: A, the B complex (including folic acid), C, D, and E.

The detailed mechanism of the action of vitamins is still hazy, although it is known that, among other things, vitamin C strengthens connective tissue and encourages formation of phagocytes, white cells that destroy invading bacteria.

It's a mistake to equate vitamins and other nutrients with drugs, however. "They are not medicines at all, and they function in an entirely different way," says one scientist. "Medicines and drugs *interfere* with metabolism; nutrients make metabolism possible."

The evidence that deficiencies or excesses of nutrients and trace elements can lead to physical and mental illness, including mood disturbances, is there for all to see, but in its often backward ways, conventional medicine has so far largely disregarded it. Conventional medicine does pay lip service to the value of vitamins, minerals, and trace elements, but most doctors naively and mistakenly tell their patients that a normal diet contains all the nutrients they need.

One reason conventional medicine has largely disregarded the role of nutrition in mental and physical health is that most medical schools do not teach clinical nutrition. Prevention is supposed to be the ideal medicine, but doctors are taught to think in terms of diseases and their supposed cures. Accordingly, they learn about vitamin-deficiency diseases—the fact that a lack of vitamin C causes scurvy, a shortage of B_1 produces beriberi, and so on. What they don't learn is that physical and mental health can be improved significantly with optimum nutrition. The doctors' misinformed advice contributes to the high rate of mood disturbances in the U.S. population.

The so-called recommended daily allowances, or RDAs, for different vitamins (widely listed on packaged foods) were formulated by the government with the disease philosophy in mind. RDAs stand for slightly more than minimum amounts of vitamins needed to protect an organism from diseases such as scurvy, but they have no bearing on optimum health.

The mistaken notion that RDAs provide sufficient nutrients for good health has taken firm hold among not only laymen but doctors, too. The misleading idea that what's readily available in the normal diet is perfectly adequate for good health has also become ingrained.

Furthermore, some people assume that living in a country as rich as the United States they get all the nutrition they need from their daily diet. But studies by government, university, and private researchers show that diet frequently to be inadequate in a variety of nutrients, including vitamins. For instance, studies at the U.S. Department of Agriculture's Experiment Station at Beltsville, Maryland, have shown that the so-called type A school lunch does not deliver one-third of those insufficient recommended daily allowances of all nutrients per meal. The U.S.D.A. had analyzed lunches from schools in various parts of the country and found them all grossly inadequate.

The deceptive nature of insufficient nutrients in the diet lies in the fact that if examined in a doctor's office the person with such marginal deficiency appears clinically normal. But because of depletion of vitamins in his tissues, such a person's metabolism—and moods—become abnormal. The individual struggles in the twilight zone between good and bad health. Irritability and general malaise set in.

The assumption that our diets contain all the nutrients we need is particularly dangerous in the kind of society we live in, where processed and preserved foods predominate while scientific nutrition is downgraded.

Just how false our assumptions are was dramatically demonstrated by Dr. Roger Williams of the University of Texas in 1970. A pioneering researcher in nutrition and health, Dr. Williams fed a group of young weanling rats commercially enriched white bread containing thiamine, riboflavin, niacin, and iron. (Milling removes those and most other nutrients, such as folic acid, vitamin B_{12}, and the trace elements. Bread manufacturers put back only those four components into the bread, however, and then label the bread "enriched." This has led Dr. Williams to remark that "enriched" flour should really be labeled "deficient.")

Another group of rats in the Williams experiment received the same bread supplemented with small amounts of minerals, vitamins, and the amino acid lysine. The rats on commercially available enriched bread fared dismally. After three months, two-thirds of them were dead and the others severely stunted.

On the other hand, most of the rats receiving the real enriched bread thrived and were still growing at the end of the experiment. Dr. Williams reported that these rats grew and developed about seven times as fast as the animals on the commercial bread.

This experiment starkly disclosed the failure of the baking and milling industry to keep abreast of the latest findings in nutrition. Unfortunately, it's far from being an isolated case; the food industry has performed dreadfully where its obligation to its customers is concerned. It has shown far more interest, for instance, in preserving the shelf life of its products with chemicals than it has in what such chemicals might be doing to our health. According to the *Wall Street Journal,* the food industry spent about $4 billion on advertising its products in 1977 alone. In a dramatic contrast, it has spent very little on real nutrition research.

Only now, years after that remarkable demonstration by Dr. Williams showing the poor nutritional qualities of "enriched" flour, is the government considering the addition of three more vitamins and three more minerals to flour.

What's more, Dr. Williams has pointed out that there is no room for complacency, because suboptimal nutrition normally prevails in nature. When organisms are very young, they are furnished with good nutrition. But after a sprout is no longer nurtured by the seed and a young animal has passed the suckling stage—or a child has reached school age—the organism no longer automatically gets what it needs to grow, and suboptimal nutrition becomes the order of the day. So the food industry has all the more reason to be concerned about the nutritional content of its products.

Yet the trends point in the opposite direction—more and more effort to make foods last longer in shipping and on the shelf, to make them look more attractive and taste better—all with chemicals. An average American already consumes an astounding five pounds of preservatives, emulsifiers, food dyes, and other similar chemicals per year, and that figure is rising constantly.

How do these chemicals affect our moods and mental health?

Dr. Feingold, the noted California pediatrician who has headed the laboratory of medical entomology at the Kaiser-Permanente Health Care Program in San Francisco, provides some troubling answers. In his recent book *Why Your Child Is Hyperactive* Dr. Feingold relates the remarkable story of a woman who came to his office one day in 1965 with her face swollen. She was suffering from acute hives and felt miserable. Tests for allergies were negative, and Dr. Feingold concluded that artificial food colors and flavors might be involved, since he had seen food additives cause hives before. He immediately placed the woman on a diet, to which she responded, and the hives vanished in about three days. Dr. Feingold found out a bit later that the woman's mental problems also disappeared. She had been in psychotherapy for two years, without visible results.

Dr. Feingold alerted his staff to be on the lookout for other cases of behavioral disturbances. Out of this program evolved the Kaiser-Permanente diet to treat hyperkinetic children, as an alternative to drugs.

Dr. Feingold does not think that food additives cause hyperkinesis but that they exacerbate it in a youngster predisposed toward hyperkinesis, the sometimes compulsive aggressive behavior that may include an uncontrolled need to touch everything. Hyperkinetic children are impulsive, excitable, and almost impossible to quiet down. They have a low tolerance for failure and frustration, a short attention span, and irregular sleep habits.

In his diet Dr. Feingold excluded all foods and drugs that were artificially dyed and flavored, as well as natural products containing salicylates. (Such natural substances act somewhat like aspirin. They are found in apricots, peaches, tomatoes, and other natural foods and can induce adverse reactions in susceptible youngsters and adults.)

The Kaiser-Permanente diet was immensely successful. Dr. Feingold prescribed this diet to the patient with hives and to hundreds of youngsters with allergies such as itching, hives, skin rashes, and asthma. The children had personality disturbances, but their behavior and learning improved after they were placed on the diet.

Dr. Feingold made the sensible suggestion that exact names of the dyes used in foods and drugs should be listed on labels to help both doctors and the general public, but this suggestion fell on deaf ears. Current labels seldom identify dyes (and other additives), stating merely that a "U.S. Certified Color" is being used.

In the view of many experts, it is possible that the burgeoning use of food additives since World War II has been responsible for the remarkable rise in the number of children displaying symptoms of hyperkinesis—the inability to remain inactive for any length of time, to concentrate, to learn as well as their intelligence would normally allow.

Many doctors have attempted to treat hyperkinetic children with tranquilizers, but that brings on problems such as depression and personality changes. There is also a suspicion that long-term use of such drugs in children leads to stunted growth. Although the behavior of some hyperkinetic children on drugs becomes more tractable, no one has ever shown that tranquilizers improve the youngsters' learning.

Criminal behavior, too, has been linked to diet, specifically to food allergies that are expressed as swellings in the brain. Although such reactions may seem rare, no one is immune from an affliction of that kind. Scientists calculate that every one of us carries anywhere from five to eight abnormal genes, and faulty genes are responsible for faulty biochemistry. Geneticists stress that for this reason the old-fashioned stigma that still clings to some genetic diseases, particularly those affecting the mind, is nonsense. Every married couple stands a 3 percent chance of bearing a genetically damaged child. The risk goes up dramatically when one carrier of a genetic disease unknowingly marries another with the same abnormality. As a result, the ratio of genetically abnormal reactions to natural and artificial substances in food appears to be quite high.

Barbara Reed, a probation officer in Cuyahoga Falls, Ohio, recently found that 82 percent of 106 offenders she tested suffered from symptoms of low blood sugar. A change to a highly nutritious diet improved the attitudes and appearances of the offenders studied. Interestingly, when Mrs. Reed's tests disclose symptoms of low blood sugar, the two municipal judges in her Ohio community can order the offender to go on a high-protein, fresh fruit and vegetable and vitamin supplement diet, replacing sweets and starches. If the offender refuses to go on this diet, his probation can be revoked.

Many offenders are found to be suffering from hypoglycemia, which may be the civilized world's most common disease. The brain is fueled by glucose, a form of sugar dissolved in the blood. Consequently, when blood sugar is lowered, the brain is affected—sometimes in such an extreme way that it causes aggressive and violent behavior. The victims of this disease are the opposites of diabetics; in hypoglycemia there is an overproduction of insulin. Carbohydrates and sugar raise the blood sugar level in response to which a hypoglycemic's oversensitive pancreas releases insulin that lowers the blood sugar content. This sends the hypoglycemic to the cupboard for more sweets, restarting the painful process. As many as one-fourth of all Americans are estimated to have some degree of hypoglycemia.

Many schizophrenics also have low blood sugar. In one study in Canada, about 90 percent of convicted schizophrenic murderers imprisoned in Saskatchewan were shown to suffer from low blood sugar or vitamin deficiencies. Some scientists have suggested that routine screening for cerebral allergies and low blood sugar should become part of admission tests to mental hospitals and prisons. The allergies and other defects could then be treated as part of a person's rehabilitation.

The way food manufacturing and distribution are organized in this country, it would be virtually impossible to do away with the excessive use of sugar and with food additives and preservatives. But there is a good reason to limit the use of sugar. Each American now consumes 120 pounds of sugar a year, compared with 12 pounds in George Washington's day. Sugar does not supply vitamins but displaces foods that do; hence, sugar contributes to malnutrition by replacing more essential nutrients. Unlike carbohydrates, which are broken down and employed in building up components of the body's cells, sugar—a relatively new food in the history of man—brings out the release of insulin, which in turn produces fatty acids that may lead to diabetes, obesity, and heart disease.

The complete elimination of food additives is unlikely, even undesirable, since some additives perform the useful function of protecting food against spoilage by such dangerous microorganisms as the botulism bacillus. But if we have to use some additives, there is a clever way to limit their access into the body's interior. Its originator is Dr. Alejandro Zaffaroni, a brilliant biochemist born in Uruguay and educated in the United States. Zaffaroni had served as executive vice-president of Syntex Corporation, the drug company that pioneered the development of the birth control pill. He left Syntex in 1968 to organize a company of his own, Alza Corporation of Palo Alto, California. This company concentrates on novel techniques of delivering drugs to the body. In the course of his scientific investigations, Zaffaroni read how certain hormones act on a cell without entering it but rather send a message into the cell's interior through the membrane. Zaffaroni asked why one couldn't apply this principle to molecules of sugar, artificial sweeteners, preservatives, and coloring agents. Let them do their job at their target organ (the tongue, in the case of sweeteners), then pass harmlessly through the stomach without entering the bloodstream and causing weight gain or possibly severe side effects, including cancer.

To put his ideas into practice, Zaffaroni organized the Dynapol Corporation to develop a number of sweeteners, coloring agents, and preservatives whose molecules are "leashed" to larger, inert molecules that will prevent the chemicals from penetrating the stomach wall. Dynapol's first products are expected on the market in the next two years or so.

Aside from Zaffaroni, a number of other outstanding thinkers recognized early on that mind and body are inseparable and interdependent and that a properly balanced nutritional environment is crucial to the realization of an individual's potential. As early as 1941, Sir Julian Huxley wrote, "Recent work has shown that vitamins and other accessory food factors have physical and mental effects far transcending what we originally thought possible." And in the early 1950s, his younger brother Aldous Huxley wrote: "The nervous system is more vulnerable than the other tissues of the body; consequently, vitamin deficiencies tend to affect the state of mind before they affect, at least in any very obvious way, the skin, bones, mucous membranes, muscles and viscera. The first result of an inadequate diet is a lowering of the efficiency of the brain as an instrument for biological survival."

But it took Linus Pauling to impart real impetus to the field of psychonutrition. A chemist who had twice won the Nobel Prize, once for chemistry and once for his efforts on behalf of world peace, Pauling became interested in medicine in 1933 when he began studying the properties of hemoglobin, the iron-containing pigment of red blood cells, and the nature of blood reactions in immunity. This research gave Pauling the idea that sickle-cell anemia was caused by abnormal hemoglobin molecules. In 1949 Pauling published a paper with his students on the molecular basis of sickle-cell anemia, formulating for the first time the concept of molecular disease.

Pauling's interest in nutrition's role in disease was stimulated in part by an experience he had as a patient. He once contracted nephritis, an inflammation of the kidneys, and his condition gradually improved under nutritional therapy—primarily a low-protein diet with supplementary vitamins, including vitamin C.

Pauling gradually became interested in vitamins' effects on schizophrenia and in 1968 published a landmark paper in the journal *Science.* Entitled "Orthomolecular Psychiatry," the paper argued that vitamins and other natural substances play a significant role in determining the mental health of a person. Dr. Pauling defined orthomolecular psychiatric therapy as the treatment of mental illness by providing an optimum molecular environment for the mind, especially an optimum molecular concentration of substances normally present in the human body. The prefix "ortho," from the Greek, means "correct" or "right," and "molecular" relates to molecules.

The fundamental idea of orthomolecular psychiatry is to bring the brain chemistry back to normal by providing those substances that occur naturally in the brain rather than depending on foreign agents that accidentally may seem to confer benefits. It is no accident, of course, that the most helpful drugs in the treatment of mental disease have been substances that resemble the brain's own neurotransmitters in their structure or that are synthetic analogues of the brain's own chemical code words of behavior, the neuropeptides.

As an example of the striking effects of dietary deficiencies in people with abnormal metabolism and how they can be ameliorated with diet, Dr. Pauling cited an inherited disease known as phenylketonuria, or PKU, a comparatively rare ailment that used to cripple its victims with severe mental retardation. Victims of PKU lack or have a low level of the enzyme phenylalanine hydroxylase, which normally oxidizes the amino acid phenylalanine, an essential ingredient of food protein. A PKU baby develops abnormal concentrations of phenylalanine in the blood and spinal fluid, which leads to damage of the central nervous system. In 1953 Horst Bickel, a German pediatrician, devised a protein-free diet that prevents the damage, or sharply reduces it, and enables most PKU victims to grow up normally. Testing for PKU in newborns is mandatory in most states now, and the diet, which costs about sixty dollars a month, is often supplied free to parents who cannot afford it.

The everyday effects of nutrients on normal people aren't as pronounced, of course, but they are as real, nonetheless. Living on a fifteen-hundred-calorie-a-day diet for six months, thirty-six normal healthy young men who had volunteered to participate in an experiment at the University of Minnesota did not become physically ill, but all suffered psychological aftereffects. Described earlier as a "highly idealistic, fun-loving, healthy group," the men turned into cynics and neurotics.

A similar study conducted with healthy women volunteers at the Mayo Clinic produced dramatic changes in the women's personalities in three months. The women became quarrelsome, hostile, and anxious. Their memories began to fail.

Even before Pauling's introduction of the term *orthomolecular psychiatry,* pioneering scientists had begun to apply some of its principles to treatment of patients with disturbed moods and minds.

The most notable practitioners of this art (in fact, their work stimulated Dr. Pauling to formulate his concept) were Dr. Abraham Hoffer and Dr. Humphry Osmond. Working in Saskatchewan, they had successfully treated schizophrenics with eighteen grams of niacin or niacinamide a day, hundreds of times the amount needed to prevent pellagra.

Pauling himself conducted successful tests on schizophrenics and now presides over the Linus Pauling Institute for Science and Medicine in Menlo Park, California. The institute's aim is to extend the orthomolecular approach to all of medicine. Developing a biochemical profile of an individual that would indicate what he or she can safely eat, what drugs the person can tolerate, and what diseases might be developing is one of the institute's goals. Unfortunately, Pauling found public funding hard to get for his unorthodox ideas and there is a real question whether the institute will survive, despite the great promise of orthomolecular medicine. The great irony is that Pauling's approach comes much closer than conventional medicine's activities to the ideal expounded by Hippocrates, the father of medicine, in his admonition to doctors to rely on nature's healing powers.

The community of orthomolecular psychiatrists has gradually expanded as the public has responded, even if conventional medicine has not. Orthomolecular psychiatrists have been particularly successful in treating hypoglycemia and the mood disturbances it causes. The treatment, which consists of vitamins and a high-protein diet, eradicates irritability, mild depression, gloomy introspection, an inability to concentrate—all symptoms of hypoglycemia. Nightmares that some hypoglycemics experience can be stopped with a high-protein bedtime snack. Pursuing a similar approach, Dr. Bernard Rimland of the Child Behavior Research Institute in San Diego showed not long ago in a study of two hundred autistic children that large doses of vitamins significantly improved the condition of two-thirds of the children.

Despite such successes, acceptance of orthomolecular psychiatry has been slow. With a pilot program involving only three counties so far, California is the only state to allow Medicaid and Medicare payments for orthomolecular treatment.

Establishment psychiatry still frowns on the field, claiming that patients who have been helped by orthomolecular psychiatry have been helped by nothing more than the vitamins' and the diets' placebo effect. Similarly, the establishment press largely ignores the field. The Huxley Institute for Biosocial Research recently sponsored a well-attended conference called Nutrient Therapy in Medicine, in New York City, and science and medical reporters from the major newspapers and magazines were conspicuous by their absence.

The Huxley Institute is the only organization in the world dedicated entirely to orthomolecular medicine. In the ten years of its existence the institute has developed programs to train physicians in the use of orthomolecular methods, to assist in the operation of the first orthomolecular clinic, and to make public the constant advances in biochemical therapy. One of its most important functions is a referral and education center through the national office (1114 First Avenue, New York, New York 10021, telephone: 212-759-9554), which receives numerous mail and telephone inquiries asking where and how orthomolecular medicine is available. Many of these calls and letters are from desperate patients and families who have suffered the agonies of mental illness and have now turned to the institute for direction and advice. The staff members always take time to discuss each caller's problem with sympathy and understanding and answer letters promptly and fully. The institute also supplies specialized material to many state health agencies, hospitals, veterans' associations, prisons, libraries, and students. Through its public education effort, the institute encourages physicians, especially psychiatrists, to investigate and adopt orthomolecular methods and to delve further into the theory and application of biochemical treatment for mental illness.

Mary Ellen Roddy, the institute's executive director, says:

> It is the Institute's conviction that this type of contact with physicians who are considering the use of orthomolecular methods in their practice is one of the most important functions of its education and referral services. The imbalance in the ratio between patients who desperately want to be treated by orthomolecular means and experienced orthomolecular physicians who offer biochemical treatment is a matter of grave concern to us. We feel it is imperative that new physicians be urged to join the ranks of orthomolecular practitioners in order that all patients receive adequate and complete orthomolecular treatment.
>
> One of the major distinctions between orthomolecular therapy and conventional therapies is the desire on the part of the orthomolecular physician to fully acquaint his patients with the nature and symptoms of his illness, and the treatment he will be given for it. The Institute and its affiliated physicians firmly believe that once a patient understands every aspect of his illness and treatment, he will be better able to work with the doctor and so take the first steps to recovery.
>
> To this end, the Institute makes available literature on schizophrenia and related disorders such as hyperactivity and learning disabilities, as well as alcoholism and drug abuse. We continually update our literature and other materials in order to keep the public informed about the latest theories and developments in the orthomolecular movement.

There are signs that the establishment is beginning to have second thoughts about its short-sighted response to nutrition and mental health. Establishment journals are, albeit reluctantly, beginning to accept scientific papers describing work in orthomolecular psychiatry.

Some establishment institutions are becoming interested in nutrition's influences on the brain—not in the effects of malnutrition on the brain, which is an old and predictable subject, but in effects of the seemingly adequate normal diet. Investigators at MIT, among other places, have recently begun to address that question.

The MIT scientists are assembling evidence showing that at least three major kinds of neurotransmitters are affected by diet. Serotonin, one such neurotransmitter, is produced in the brain from the amino acid tryptophan, which comes from digested protein and is carried to the brain by the bloodstream.

But to get tryptophan into the brain takes some doing, the MIT scientists discovered, since it can't penetrate the blood-brain barrier that protects the brain from many foreign substances. Tryptophan can cross the blood-brain barrier only with the aid of a "transport protein." But at least eight other amino acids compete for the services of these transport molecules. Accordingly, the amount of tryptophan in the blood must exceed the volume of the other amino acids in order to get into the brain. The reason a big carbohydrate meal makes a person sleepy is that carbohydrates release relatively large concentrations of tryptophan, which then synthesizes serotonin, which in turn has soothing and inhibiting effects.

On the other hand, a sharp decrease in serotonin concentrations makes a rat (and probably a human) more sensitive to pain. Some psychotic illnesses may thus result from a relative deficiency of tryptophan in the diet, scientists suggest. Some studies show that depressed people may benefit from eating foods containing tryptophan. These include carbohydrates as well as milk and cheese products. "The idea that normal diets can affect brain metabolism is becoming established," concluded *Science,* the journal of the American Association for the Advancement of Science, recently.

At MIT, Richard Wurtman and his associates are beginning studies of normal human volunteers to pinpoint more precisely how different components of diet influence moods. Wurtman wrote recently that "the simple choice between eating an apple and a chicken leg may determine how much serotonin the brain will make during the postprandial period, and a week of luncheon omelettes would probably elevate acetylcholine levels in the basal ganglia." (Acetylcholine is a brain-signal transmitter associated with mood swings in mania and depression.)

The emphasis in the MIT work on normal people is important because it is not only obviously mentally distressed individuals who can benefit from larger doses of specific vitamins and other nutrients. Milder mental disorders such as anxiety neuroses are common in the population at large, as about one in every twenty Americans displays such neurotic symptoms as fatigue, frequent loss of appetite, and dizziness.

These people may need an extra supply of vitamin C, which is used up in large amounts by an organism under stress. (In some still unknown ways, the lactate metabolism in those suffering from mood disturbances appears to be involved; infusion of lactate into volunteers has produced anxiety attacks. These attacks can be counteracted by administering calcium, however.)

As did the guinea pig, certain monkeys, a few birds, and a type of bat, man lost the ability to make vitamin C in his body and must therefore receive it from outside sources. The U.S. Recommended Daily Allowance for vitamin C—forty milligrams per day for children, fifty-five for women, and sixty for men—is somewhat more than the amount needed to avoid visible symptoms of scurvy. Many scientists, including Dr. Pauling, have questioned the official RDA for vitamin C and other vitamins as well. They have pointed out that animals that synthesize vitamin C in their bodies would be unlikely to synthesize more of the vitamin than they needed for optimal health. Yet, proportionate to their weight, these animals make far greater amounts of the vitamin than the RDA prescribed for human use. If an animal weighed 154 pounds, the weight of an average man, it would make from two to nineteen grams of vitamin C per day. This suggests that similar amounts may be near optimum for man. Mammals that have been studied include mice weighing less than an ounce and goats nearly as big as people. A mouse makes the equivalent of nineteen grams of vitamin C (again, calculated to 154 pounds of body weight), a goat, thirteen grams per day. Dr. Pauling views this as evidence that the optimum intake for man is far larger than the RDA, perhaps even 100 times as large, or about five grams a day. But individual biochemical variability is so great that the range may well be from 250 milligrams to ten grams. Dr. Pauling estimates, therefore, that for many people one to two grams per day is about the optimum rate of ingestion.

There is other experimental evidence that man most likely needs more vitamin C than the RDAs prescribe. For instance, some years ago Dr. Williams obtained evidence that young guinea pigs need for good health and development at least 100 times as much vitamin C as they need to protect them from scurvy. Human beings may respond similarly.

Dr. Pauling and his wife have each been taking six grams of vitamin C a day for years and report an increased feeling of well-being and a striking decrease in the number and severity of colds they have caught.

For all practical purposes, vitamin C is nontoxic and is so described in the medical literature. Some people have taken as much as forty grams a day for months without ill effects, and others have consumed as much as one hundred grams—a quarter of a pound—a day for days, also without harm. But some people do develop diarrhea if they take vitamin C on an empty stomach in gram quantities. Accordingly, Dr. Pauling recommends that the vitamin usually be taken at the end of a meal. Most other vitamins (being foods, not drugs) are equally nontoxic—if consumed in sensibly small amounts, of course.*

To be sure, undue emphasis on any single nutrient to the detriment of others smacks of food faddism, which is as bad as neglect of nutrition as a factor in mental and physical health. It is imperative for any sensible person not to succumb to any food fad but to maintain a balanced intake of vitamins and other nutrients. One reason vitamin C has figured so prominently in nutrition is that it has been studied

*Consumed in excessive amounts, certain vitamins can be more dangerous than others. The journal of the American Medical Association in October 1977 reported the case of a four-year-old boy suffering from high fever and extreme irritability. The vitamin A level in the boy's blood was found to be ten times normal. Investigation revealed that the boy's grandmother owned a health food store and that the child's nursery school teachers had observed him bringing a bottle of vitamin tablets to school and eating them continuously. The AMA journal warned in an editorial that "when consumed in excessive amounts, almost any vitamin can cause mischief." It singled out the fat-soluble vitamins A and D as being particularly noxious—in excessive amounts.

more than other vitamins. For instance, had as much knowledge been accumulated about vitamin E—which is still something of an orphan of the vitamin family, as its exact role is not clearly defined—it would have figured much more prominently on the list of suggested nutrients.

Researchers warn about the danger of overemphasizing a single nutrient or group of nutrients. "We tend to look for magic bullets—but there are no magic bullets," says Dr. Emanuel Cheraskin, a University of Alabama investigator into nutrition and health.

Except for cases of pronounced genetic disease, a deficiency of any single nutrient is believed to be uncommon in mental illness. The relationship between the lack of a vitamin and mental illness is not as clear-cut in many cases as is the lack of niacinamide with pellagra. Deficiencies in combinations of vitamins and other nutrients and their depletion from tissues can cause depressed moods and lead to more serious symptoms of mental illness.

In studying groups of people who display superior health—in particular certain doctors, dentists, and their spouses—Dr. Cheraskin found that those who have the fewest symptoms of mental or physical disturbances avoid refined sugar and refined carbohydrates such as refined flour and rice, and consume vitamins in doses many times those listed as RDAs.

In a recent book he coauthored, *Psychodiatetics,* Dr. Cheraskin stressed the need for everyone to eat foods that help resist disease—foods that contain proteins, minerals, and essential fats such as meats, seafood, fowl, and cheese—and to avoid sugar, white flour, and food preservatives. With this diet Dr. Cheraskin and his associates have successfully treated many patients who complained of constant irritability, anxiety, insomnia, and other malign moods and irrational behavior.

Dr. Cheraskin added in a recent interview that even the best diet is not quite enough in itself for optimum health. Other factors besides adequate nutrition are involved in successful mood control. Lack of exercise—a daily half-hour walk will do—is one such factor.

"We've lost our mobility," says Dr. Cheraskin, "and that is doing us in, among other things. One could take a group of fat women," he adds, "and walk them 30 minutes every day for 10 days and by the tenth day the circumference of the average upper arm would be less, suggesting the constitutional effect."

Lack of exposure to sunlight is another negative factor. Sunlight's beneficial effect lies partly in its stimulating the pituitary through photoreceptors in the eyes. "Biologically speaking," says Dr. Cheraskin, "most of us haven't been outdoors in the last 20 or 30 years. Spend an hour each sunny day walking outside without sunglasses."

Some scientists have speculated that lack of sunlight in Sweden and other northern countries may be responsible in part for the high suicide rate because not enough vitamin D, which is synthesized by the sun's rays in the human body, is being produced in the people involved. Vitamin D is essential for the assimilation of calcium, which in turn is vital to the normal functioning of the brain.

How can we select the best food components we need for the best mental and physical health? Some years ago my wife, Gwen, while pregnant and consequently more conscious than usual of nutrition, discovered an easy way to stay on a balanced diet, by making it colorful —literally. A color-coded diet, she found, ensured a supply of all the nutrients needed by the body. She made certain that each day's meals included foods of the colors yellow, white, red, green, orange, and brown.

Sweet potatoes, carrots, squash, pumpkins, hard cheese, and butter are all yellow and are all sources of vitamin A, which aids in the building and growth of body cells.

White represents milk, bread, and eggs, yielding calcium, needed for bone and teeth building, and vitamin D, the lack of which leads to serious bone changes and the presence of which helps to build resistance to infection and to keep the skin healthy. Vitamin D is also essential for assimilation of calcium, which is vital to normal brain function.

Leafy green vegetables are a rich source of vitamins A and C. Vitamin C not only prevents scurvy but is essential for healthy blood vessels and sound bones and teeth. Without it, sore gums, hemorrhages under the skin, and general fatigue result.

Orange represents citrus fruit, source of vitamin C.

Red stands for meat, which supplies protein to rebuild body tissue.

Brown represents bread, a source of energy-supplying carbohydrates.

Many other items could and should be added to this simplified diet. To cite just a few: tomatoes, raw cabbage, and salad greens for additional vitamin C and A; liver, oysters, dried fruit, and whole or enriched grains and cereals as a source of iron; and potatoes, beets, onions, celery, eggplant, corn, parsnips, cucumbers, and white turnips as a source of various vitamins and minerals.

There is also such a thing as "body wisdom," of course. Since we depend for our existence on food, a gross deficiency in one or more of its components sometimes signals that it's time to have that component. That's why children deficient in calcium have been known to hungrily attack pieces of chalk in school.

But how can an individual exercise such body wisdom in trying to keep all those chemical additives *out* of his food, when most of it comes with additives? Obviously, this is an extremely difficult task—what person has time to read and analyze the fine print on every package of food he buys?

As Dr. Feingold has suggested, a helpful development would be to identify packaged food that is free of additives with a special symbol. So far, industry has largely resisted such suggestions. Instead, it has sought to discredit Dr. Feingold's findings about additives' harmful effects.

The only way this problem will be solved is through public pressure on food manufacturers and government authorities. Such pressure by concerned mothers recently led to the removal of sugar from baby food, which was there to make the food more appealing to mothers as they tasted it. And some manufacturers now offer breakfast cereals fortified with vitamins and other nutrients.

Similar pressure from parents' groups is bound to force food manufacturers to change their shortsighted policy on food additives. Hyperkinesis has become not only an American but a worldwide problem, too. Dr. Feingold calls it "probably one of the most critical problems of our contemporary culture." He adds that behavioral disturbances and learning disabilities with their various unpleasant consequences (truancy, vandalism, juvenile delinquency, and crime) are on the rise, "presenting one of the most disturbing social situations of our times. I believe these problems are in great measure related to our food culture. My hypothesis linking food additives to behavior and learning disabilities is only one band in a broad spectrum of social and health difficulties related to our food supply. Resolution of the situation cannot be mandated or legislated. Its correction is contingent upon public involvement, which can only be realized through public awareness and education."

So effective has Dr. Feingold's diet been in salvaging thousands of children from disturbed homes, failure at school, and a zombielike existence on conventional behavior-modifying drugs that more than one hundred parents' groups, known as Feingold Associations, have sprung up around the country. These groups allow parents to exchange their experiences as well as menus, recipes, and lists of permissible foods that are available in the local supermarkets. The associations are beginning to influence doctors through the dramatic responses of children to dietary intervention. The parents' groups also provide gatherings for the children, which permit them to interact and that also helps them. The Feingold Associations are so new that they are frequently administered from the president's home. Many aren't listed yet in local telephone books but usually can be located through local newspapers or radio and television stations.

Dr. Ruth Sabo, a young psychologist and founder of the Feingold Association for the Albany–Troy, New York, area, typically reports "terrific improvement" in more than half of the hyperkinetic and retarded children treated with the Feingold diet. The results of Feingold groups are even better than Dr. Feingold himself attained, and he reported a positive response in 30 to 40 percent of the hyperkinetic children treated.

Association members and other interested individuals—some grown-ups are susceptible to the deleterious effects of food additives, too—have devised strategies of buying products that contain no additives. Of particular concern are artificial colors, flavors, and preservatives, especially BHT (butylated hydroxytoluene) and BHA (butylated hydroxyanisole), found in butter, margarines, bread, potato chips, and in cooking oils and fats. The buying strategies include following the lists prepared by the associations. Some additivefree products can be bought at local supermarkets, and some people supplement their purchases at natural food stores. Some also buy imported hams, cookies, crackers, fish, and soups, which are often additivefree. Some purchasers wind up spending somewhat more for their food, but some, Dr. Sabo reports, actually save five to ten dollars a week because, ironically, manufacturers' high-priced, high-profit items are usually packed with additives. Not *all* American food companies rely on additives; some manufacturers have never used them yet have thrived, raising the question as to why other manufacturers use these chemicals to excess.

Although local supermarkets have been fighting the Feingold Associations—some supermarket executives have exerted pressure on the advertising departments of newspapers not to run stories about harm caused by food additives—it will be more and more difficult for the food industry to claim that all additives are harmless. Recent research at the University of Maryland, for instance, hints at devastating findings to come. This particular research has shown that tiny amounts of additives have negative effects on the electrical potential of the neuronal membrane, meaning that they cause distortions in perception and hence behavior.

It will take some time, of course, before public pressure causes food manufacturers to retreat. Meanwhile, the smart consumer will stay away as much as possible from processed foods, foods filled with additives, and fad diets that neglect to point out that supplementary vitamins and other nutrients should be taken on any such diet. (On a low-calorie diet of one thousand or fewer calories a day, an individual automatically consumes 50 percent fewer vitamins as a result of his reduced caloric intake, a fact generally overlooked by both dieters and doctors.)

In addition to dieters, others who require vitamin supplements are finicky eaters, alcoholics, smokers, and women on the birth control pill. It has been shown that such women have reduced blood levels of vitamins B_1, B_2, B_6, folic acid, and B_{12}.

The answer to the so-called marginal deficiency state, a widespread affliction in America, is not to succumb to a food fad but to achieve a well-balanced diet, to exercise, and to get enough sunlight. The key word is *balance.* The sooner we achieve it, the better off all of us will be, physically and mentally.

PART II

This Newer, Higher Brain

CHAPTER FOUR

Psychopharmacology: Fighting Depression

"The dawn of the 21st Century may witness an end to the scourge of madness."

—Dr. Norman Garmezy,
professor of psychology,
University of Minnesota

In the still mysterious world of mental illness there are beginning to appear some promising flashes of insight into both the nature of the mind's disorders and more effective ways of treating them. These advances are being generated by a burgeoning assault on the biochemistry and genetics of mental disturbances. In searching for causes of psychiatric diseases, scientists have begun to study the alterations inside the cell as well as the subcellular region. Their search has already revealed some of the biochemical and genetic mechanisms involved in the malfunctions of the mind and offers hints that some outside influences on behavior are impressed early in an organism's development as biological codes in that deepest machinery of life. Furthermore, the biological "attack" is now beginning to pay off in terms of more precise and reliable diagnoses of the still vague and varied symptoms of mental disease. The work now in progress can be expected to lay bare some of the deep causes of mental illness, vastly improving the treatment of these maladies through direct action on the structure or function of the organism.

All this is a far cry from Sigmund Freud, analysts' couches, and the baroque and musty world of the id, super ego, and libido. Freud himself, with characteristic foresight, predicted that many behavior manifestations would ultimately be traced to biochemical bases. But Freud, rooted in his time's primitive biology, decided to look at the psychological side of mental illness because he felt that was the only way he could treat patients then. In the process he introduced new dimensions into psychiatry; for instance, the role of unconscious motivations and the importance of childhood experience. Says the neurophysiologist Seymour Kety, a brilliant leader of the new biological psychiatry: "We must remember until Freud came along psychiatry was abysmally simplistic. Psychiatry was sharing the general conviction of the day, reinforced by the discoveries that came from the germ theory of disease, that mental disorders had a single cause which could be determined by looking long enough through the microscope."

What's going on in psychiatry today also involves looking at the brain or at what's going on in the brain, but on a different, much finer level and with vastly improved tools and techniques. Psychoanalysis has not been abandoned, and environmental influences have not been discarded, but psychoanalysis is taking on new forms. It is being used in group therapy, for instance, to treat couples with marital problems or groups of schizophrenic families—but in conjunction with drugs. The role of the psychoanalyst as the chief figure in psychiatry is rapidly declining. The people making the important contributions to psychiatry today often aren't even psychiatrists. John Olney in the Washington University department of psychiatry in Saint Louis typifies the new trend. As it happens, he is a psychiatrist, but he is also a highly trained specialist in electron microscopy, engaged in studies of animal and human brains. In the same department, Ferris N. Pitts, Jr., associate professor of psychiatry, uses a couch in his office not for psychoanalysis but to administer an anxiety-producing substance to volunteers. Where psychoanalysts once reigned as university psychiatry department heads, more often than not one will now find individuals who are trained specialists in biochemistry or another science as well as in psychiatry.

Psychoanalysis went into a tailspin decline with the massive arrival of mind-affecting drugs in the mid-1950s. The effectiveness of psychoanalysis had never been too impressive; its lengthy and expensive sessions furthermore confined its use to the relatively affluent. Drugs, in contrast, could be applied en masse. For more than two decades now, tranquilizers and other drugs have helped maintain a decline in the resident patient population in this country's state and county mental hospitals.

Drugs that affect the mind often do work better in conjunction with psychotherapy or counseling. This need not involve a professional psychiatrist, it is now recognized. A talk with a minister, a priest, or simply a friend who will listen may do just as well and will cost nothing. The current drugs may have some limitations, of course. None cure mental illness; they only suppress its symptoms, and many can cause serious side effects. Smith, Kline and French, the maker of Thorazine, probably the most widely used tranquilizer, lists fourteen observed and potential side effects for the drug, including seizures, lowered blood pressure, and skin disorders. But the psychotropic drugs did open up the great biochemical arena of the mind to impressive new investigations, which can be expected to produce safer and more effective chemicals.

Most of the significant current work, which is in the fields of mania and depression, involves studies of the so-called biogenic amines noradrenaline, serotonin, and dopamine. (Noradrenaline, also known as norepinephrine, is the precursor of adrenaline, the well known "fight or flight" hormone that mobilizes sugar into the bloodstream in emergencies.) All are substances manufactured by the body, all are involved as chemical transmitters or modulators of bioelectrical signals in the brain (see Chapters 1 and 2). Scientists' efforts are concentrated mainly on mania and depression because these conditions are much easier to diagnose and define than is schizophrenia. All three are classified as psychoses, conditions much more serious than neuroses. A neurotic often recognizes his trouble and may be able to contribute to his recovery, but a psychotic often will have lost some or all contact with reality.

Manics have periods of elation, a few depressed patients stay depressed all the time, and manic-depressives may have alternating periods of gloom and glow. In more severe cases manic-depressives are psychotic—they have lost contact with reality.

Some interesting research is also being done on schizophrenia. A schizophrenic usually has disturbances of thought as well as of mood and behavior. The numerous varieties of what is believed to be schizophrenia, and some symptoms overlapping between it and both mania and depression, make diagnosis extremely difficult. Karl Menninger has likened the diagnosis of types of schizophrenias to the casual way little girls name their dolls. Another reason more research is aimed at manic-depressive disorders than at schizophrenia is that the former are more consistently amenable to drug treatment, which enables investigators to set up better-controlled tests on both people and animals.

The story of how scientists became interested in noradrenaline and how they got some imaginative ideas about the possible biochemical causes of schizophrenia goes back to the beginning of psychopharmacology's golden age when fantastic new drugs began to tumble into psychiatrists' laps. First, in 1943, came LSD (lysergic acid diethylamide), the extremely potent drug that produces symptoms and behavior resembling certain psychoses. LSD was discovered by accident when Albert Hofmann, an organic chemist who worked for Sandoz, A.G., was "seized by a peculiar sensation of vertigo and restlessness," as he recalled later. "Objects, as well as the shape of my associates in the laboratory, appeared to undergo optical changes. . . . In a dreamlike state, I left for home, where an irresistible urge to lie down overcame me. . . . With my eyes closed, fantastic pictures of extraordinary plasticity and intensive color seemed to surge toward me. After two hours this state gradually wore off." Hofmann decided that he had somehow ingested some of the compound on which he happened to be working, a derivative of ergot, a fungus that grows on rye. He then took one-quarter milligram of the drug, with even more spectacular results. LSD wasn't the first hallucinogen, but its ability to produce strange visions with fantastically small amounts (as little as twenty micrograms, for example, the equivalent of one-third of a grain of salt) was unprecedented.

The extraordinary potency of LSD aroused the interest of biochemists and other scientists, who were particularly intrigued by the fact that a chemical substance could produce a state somewhat akin to schizophrenia. "It showed that a minute trace of a substance can change a person's thinking and perception," says Kety. "One often gets a feeling when talking to a schizophrenic that he's being acted upon by something like that. It's only a hunch. But a lot of the best scientific theories were originally based on such hunches or insights."

By the late forties, American and Italian researchers, in separate investigations, had become intrigued by a substance that was to make LSD seem even more interesting—serotonin. It had been known to exist in minute amounts in the blood, but now it was found in body tissues as well. In 1953 Martha Volk in Britain found that serotonin was detectable in the brain, concentrated in its limbic system, an area deep in the brain that governs emotional states. The story became more exciting when in 1954 D. W. Wooley in the United States and John Gattum in England found LSD to be a potent antagonist of serotonin. They observed that when serotonin made the intestine contract, a minute dose of LSD put into the laboratory bath would stop the contraction.

At this point some scientists began to speculate that LSD might cause psychosislike symptoms by inhibiting serotonin in the brain. They suspected serotonin of acting as a signal transmitter or modulator. But just how serotonin acted—whether it facilitated or hindered the flow of brain-nerve impulses—wasn't entirely clear.

These questions become still more interesting in the mid-fifties when serotonin became implicated in mania and depression. This finding was related to the discovery of reserpine, an extract of the dried root of *Rauwolfia serpentina,* used for centuries in India to treat epilepsy, insomnia, snake bites, and many other ills. Reserpine was first used by modern Western doctors to treat high blood pressure. They noticed its tranquilizing effect on many patients and found that it produced severe depression in some. Here again, change in mood was related to serotonin. In 1955 Bernard Brodie, Parkhurst Shore, and their colleagues at the U.S. National Heart Institute discovered that reserpine caused a remarkable depletion of serotonin in the brain. In some cases the compound disappeared almost entirely.

By this time doctors had another amazing drug in their hands. Iproniazid had been synthesized in the United States to treat tuberculosis. Like reserpine, it not only changed behavior but also made changes related to the amount of serotonin in the brain. When given in even small doses, iproniazid made tubercular patients dance in the hospital halls. Mental-health researchers, their curiosity aroused, found that iproniazid lifted the level of serotonin in the brain and elevated the mood of the mentally ill.

To have stumbled within a few years on two drugs with completely opposite effects was remarkable. "Here was a wonderful thing," remarks Kety. "A drug that depressed, lowered serotonin. A drug that elevated mood, raised serotonin." It was wonderful because biochemists now had a clue as to what might be happening in the brain chemically when someone became depressed. Besides, they could now experiment on animals by manipulating the two types of drugs.

It soon became clear that changes in the level of serotonin were not the entire explanation of mania and depression. It was found that the new drugs caused similar changes in the noradrenaline and dopamine levels. The research emphasis now shifted to noradrenaline because it yielded more provocative results.

Out of these dramatic explorations has grown the so-called catecholamine hypothesis of mood disorders, the most coherent and best-supported theory about the biochemistry of depression. Catecholamines are a group of biogenic amines including noradrenaline and dopamine. In the early 1960s Joseph Schildkraut, director of the neuropsychopharmacology laboratory at the Massachusetts Mental Health Center, probably did more than anyone else to organize the evidence. The hypothesis holds that noradrenaline levels are low at certain brain sites in depressed people and high in those suffering from mania. Noradrenaline apparently affects the activity of some brain-cell systems, systems that may serve as mood regulators.

The catecholamine hypothesis rests on pioneering investigations of what happens to noradrenaline in the brain. A large amount of this ground-breaking work was accomplished in the Laboratory of Clinical Science of the National Institute of Mental Health in Bethesda, Maryland, by Kety, Julius Axelrod, Irwin Kopin, and others. Kety, then director of the laboratory, had the feeling that what happens to noradrenaline in the brain is critical. He commissioned the radiology laboratory to synthesize a few milligrams of noradrenaline tagged with a highly radioactive tritium. After injecting this substance into the brains of animals, Axelrod proceeded to predict and verify its metabolic pathway in the body and its storage and release in various neurons or nerve cells.

The highest concentrations of noradrenaline occur in the hypothalamus, a region of the brain associated with control of the emotions. Using mind-influencing drugs as a strategic research tool, biochemists have further established how noradrenaline works in the brain.

The biochemists used two main classes of antidepressant drugs, both of which apparently intensify noradrenaline's action at receptor sites between neurons. The two types of drugs work in different ways but lead to the same result. One class of chemicals, known as monoamine oxidase inhibitors, depresses the activity of the enzyme monoamine oxidase, which normally inactivates noradrenaline released from the storage granules at neuronal junctures. The second category of antidepressants (such as imipramine, for example) inhibits the return of noradrenaline to the storage granules after it has been used as a signal transmitter. In both cases more noradrenaline becomes available at receptor sites, something like freight cars jammed into a railroad switch yard.

These "freight" cars are loaded with "happy" merchandise, for an increase in the amounts of noradrenaline at nerve endings lifts moods. Cocaine, which Freud was one of the first to recognize as a euphoriant, shares some properties with imipramine-type drugs and, not surprisingly, produces pleasurable feelings. Similarly, the widely used amphetamine stimulants (Benzedrine, Dexadrine, and so on) appear to discharge stored noradrenaline from the nerve endings in the brain, thus leading to better feelings.

Conversely, depletion of noradrenaline makes moods dip. Lithium salts, effective in treating mania, impede the release of noradrenaline. Lowered amounts of this biogenic amine also explain why some women who take birth control pills are often depressed, lethargic, or irritable. A few years ago scientists from the University of North Carolina reported that such women with mood disturbances showed alteration in metabolism of noradrenaline and other catecholamines. This suggests that hormones influence a person's mood through the biogenic amines. In another project, a group of University of Washington investigators showed that the behavior effects of LSD in rabbits depend on the levels of noradrenaline in their brains: the more noradrenaline, the more excited and active the rabbits. The sustained therapeutic effect of electroshock, still the most effective treatment for depression, also appears to take place through noradrenaline. Recent tests on animals show that electroshock produces a long-lasting increase in the amounts of noradrenaline in their brains. Somewhat to their surprise, scientists found that electroshock administered to the feet of animals also boosts noradrenaline levels in the brain. This raises the question whether electric shock could not be replaced by stress of other types administered in gentler ways to cause a discharge of brain noradrenaline to improve patients. A Chicago scientific team reports such improvement by imposing stresses of various types on depressed patients. Some investigators claim to have gotten improvement in their hospitalized depressed patients by assigning them seemingly unpleasant chores such as mopping floors. This activity becomes emotionally soothing, something many women have known for a long time. Kety suggests that stress of any kind sets off a great flow of steroid hormones that in turn energize an enzyme that synthesizes noradrenaline.

A deficiency in noradrenaline metabolism could come about through impairment of its binding and storage, increased release of noradrenaline inside the cells, and an accompanying increased destruction of the neurohormone by the enzyme that inhibits it, as well as decreased sensitivity to noradrenaline at receptor sites. Patients suffering from different varieties of depression may be reflecting such different mechanisms, all of which lead to depletion of noradrenaline at crucial sites.

It hasn't been easy to discover some of these things, because investigators of the biochemistry of mental illness have to cope with a number of serious obstacles. For one thing, there isn't really a good animal model of depression, anxiety, or another mental disease that would mirror precisely such conditions in man. Furthermore, the human brain is not only the most complex and inaccessible organ but is also protected by the blood-brain barrier. Kety says, "We know that if you give radioactive sodium and then kill the animal in twenty minutes, the sodium will have left the blood vessels and gone into the extracellular fluid of every organ in the body except the brain. In the brain it will stay within the blood vessels." The current concept is that the brain's glial cells, which encircle the capillaries, act as the blood-brain barrier. Somehow, these cells recognize what is useful to the brain and what isn't. Useful substances such as oxygen, certain amino acids, or glucose are allowed to pass into the brain, but a potentially toxic substance is generally kept out.

Among the substances blocked by the barrier are noradrenaline and serotonin. But L-dopa, a precursor of both dopamine and noradrenaline, does penetrate the blood-brain barrier when given in large doses. This recent discovery has brought about effective and dramatic treatment of Parkinsonism, a muscle-disorganizing nerve malady linked to a dopamine deficit in the brain. Dopamine is concentrated in portions of the brain that control motor, or muscle, activity. Parkinsonism resembles a form of schizophrenia called catatonia.

Giving depressed patients L-dopa has recently yielded direct support for the catecholamine hypothesis. Such patients, after receiving good-sized doses of L-dopa, react as the hypothesis predicts: L-dopa produces anger in most patients studied and a high incidence of mania in manic-depressives. Similarly, in animals large doses of L-dopa reverse the sluggishness and apathy induced by reserpine and build up the volume of noradrenaline.

To obviate the blood barrier, scientists at the National Institute of Mental Health devised a technique for injecting radioactive amines directly into an animal's lateral ventricles, fluid-filled chambers lodged alongside the midline of the brain. These chambers are inside the blood-brain barrier. This technique paved the way for tracing the effects of psychoactive drugs on noradrenaline metabolism directly inside a living brain.

In a few limited instances, human brains have become accessible to similar studies. Patients at the National Institutes of Health Clinical Center in Bethesda, Maryland, with inoperable brain tumors receive drugs through catheters inserted into their lateral ventricles. Through the catheters medications are gently pumped into the brain, and cerebral spinal fluid can be withdrawn for analysis. With the patients' consent, scientists are injecting tracer amounts of various biogenic amines and their precursors into the brains and drawing samples for assay as the patients' moods shift. This work hasn't progressed far enough yet for the investigators to come to any firm conclusions.

It is highly important to try to assess the fate of biogenic amines in human and animal brains directly. The reason is that the blood-brain barrier for all practical purposes also prevents many key substances such as noradrenaline from *leaving* the brain. Since the human brain generally is inaccessible to direct experimentation, scientists have been forced to measure the amounts of noradrenaline and its metabolites in urine and blood. Most of these substances come not from the brain but from the peripheral nervous system, where noradrenaline is indisputably the transmitter agent of nerve impulses.

From these measurements many investigators have obtained support for the catecholamine hypothesis. Until recently, the unanswered question was in what molecular form the breakdown products of noradrenaline left the brain. Within the past year, scientists have moved closer to answering that question. Independently and simultaneously, two teams of investigators, at the National Institute of Mental Health and the University of Illinois, identified a compound called MHPG as the major product of metabolic change of noradrenaline. The substance was found in the brains of test animals as well as in their urine.

Looking for MHPG in both depressed and manic patients, scientists have found its levels consistently lower in depressed people than in normal ones and higher in manic patients. There is a good chance that MHPG will turn out to be a far more precise and direct indicator of activity in the brain's adrenergic nerve cells—neurons activated by noradrenaline—than any other metabolic product. This finding is now being employed as the basis for developing biochemical tests for routine use by psychiatrists to diagnose varieties of depression, since MHPG levels differ in patients suffering from different types of mental distress. Significantly, MHPG levels fall in people with a variety of depressive symptoms, even in those in whom readings of noradrenaline metabolic products in the past appeared somewhat confusing and contradictory. Patients with agitated depression typically express their worries through constant hand wringing, pacing the floor, and similar acts.

There is still disagreement among psychiatrists whether depressed patients can really be divided into the two traditional major diagnostic categories: those with endogenous (internally caused) or exogenous (externally caused) depression. This separation receives some support from findings by psychiatric geneticists as well as from the results of drug and electroshock treatment. Such treatment appears to be more effective against depressions that seem to have lives of their own. Treatment works less well when a person becomes depressed because of external circumstances. External stress apparently influences somewhat different biochemical pathways.

Schildkraut likens a person with internally caused depression to "a blown light bulb in which the filament has to be repaired. A person with an externally caused depression, on the other hand, is like a perfect light bulb—only there isn't enough juice."

The early experiments with LSD suggested that serotonin may contribute to mental illness in a rather spectacular way: as raw material for a hallucinogen. In 1961 Axelrod found high concentrations of an enzyme, indoleamine-N-methyltransferase, in the lungs of rabbits. This enzyme can convert serotonin to bufotenine. It can also turn tryptamine, an amino acid by-product, into dimethyltryptamine (DMT). Both bufotenine and DMT are hallucinogens, somewhat similar to LSD. The meaning of this startling discovery is that the body's own biochemical machinery can manufacture psychosis-producing "poisons." After his discovery, Axelrod wrote, "Thus the body has all the biochemical machinery to convert normally-occurring compounds to psychomimetic [psychosis-producing] metabolites."

Arnold J. Mandell, then at the University of California's Irvine campus, figured that such hallucinogens might be produced when the levels of biogenic amines in the brain became elevated by antidepressant drugs. He treated young chicks with one such drug and found the two hallucinogens in the chicks' brains. (The effect of those substances on chicks was to make them drop their wings for two or three hours.)

Excited about their discovery, Mandell and his associates engaged in a hectic, night-and-day hunt for Axelrod's enzyme. They found it two months later at the nerve endings in the chicks' brain cells, where one neuron communicates with another. This marked the first time the enzyme had been found in the brain of any animal.

Mandell describes his discovery as being both scary and thrilling, the former because of its staggering implications (hinted at before by Axelrod and others) that at least some forms of mental disorders may be induced when the human body itself makes psychotogenic "poisons." It was a thrilling discovery because an explanation of and possibly effective treatment for such scrious disorders as paranoid schizophrenia might be forthcoming.

In very small doses, all the hallucinogens—LSD, mescaline, bufotenine, DMT, and others—produce not hallucinations but periods of euphoria and hyperactivity. But in larger doses the drugs become toxic and produce delusions, hallucinations, and psychosis. One set of stimulants, the amphetamines, can call forth in some people what is known as amphetamine psychosis, a state difficult to distinguish from paranoid schizophrenia. This is characterized by delusions of grandeur or persecution and by hallucinations. It was this type of drug that produced hallucinogens in the chicks. What Mandell suggests is that something —perhaps a sudden, emotionally painful experience—mobilizes normally unused enzymes and sends them along normally untraveled metabolic pathways in a person's brain to produce hallucinogens.

The secret hope of a big breakthrough pushed Mandell and his coworkers into a search for Axelrod's enzyme in the human brain. Working with a team of brain surgeons at UCLA who were excising portions of brain to cure epileptics, thus making available rare brain material for analysis, Mandell and his associates in 1973 found the enzyme in the human brain.

A number of scientists have since suggested the fascinating possibility that persons genetically predisposed to mental disorders may respond to stress by producing too much DMT. In small quantities, DMT may act as a euphoriant, just as hallucinogenic drugs do in small doses. DMT may thus be the stuff pleasant thoughts are made of. It may also have a lot to do with carrying from neuron to neuron information that relates to imagination, dreaming, daydreaming, and formation of individual personality. Too much DMT, though, would act as a psychic poison, especially in people genetically predisposed to its excessive production.

The search is already on for chemicals that might block the excessive formation of such hallucinogens, a search spurred on by an earlier finding of Arnold Friedhoff from New York University medical school of a mescalinelike compound in the urine of schizophrenics. Mescaline was originally derived from peyote, a cactus used by American Indians in religious ceremonies. At least two drug companies, Merck and Sandoz, are searching for nontoxic inhibitors of the transmethylation process believed to be involved in the manufacture of the hallucinogens in the brain. In this process, groups of atoms in the catecholamines are believed to be substituted by other atoms, producing the hallucinogen mescaline as a methylated derivative of the catecholamines.

The transmethylation-psychosis hypothesis is not easily explained in terms of what is known about the brain's ability to protect itself against bombardment by strange substances. It isn't only the blood-brain barrier that protects it. The brain has a mechanism, a receptor level, that helps it adjust to strange substances that do penetrate the blood-brain barrier. For instance, the same dose of LSD taken on consecutive days becomes less and less effective. Obviously, this compensation breaks down somehow when people are disturbed, because they can remain disturbed for a long, long time.

Although a lot of pieces have fallen into place lately to support the catecholamine hypothesis, no one argues that noradrenaline or its relatives can explain everything about depressions or manias. "This is a segment of the story, but it isn't the whole pie," says one researcher. Schildkraut and Kety have written that any comprehensive explanation of physiology of mood would have to take into account many other biochemical, physiological, and psychological factors.

Among such factors still poorly understood are the interrelationships between hormones, electrolytes, and postulated brain impulse transmitters or regulators such as noradrenaline. Electrolytes are substances such as sodium, potassium, and calcium that in solution are capable of conducting an electric current. They play a vital role in nerve impulse generation and transmission. Potassium ions are concentrated inside a neuron, sodium ions outside. An electrochemical equilibrium is maintained between the two by an electric potential in the membrane of the neuron. This keeps sodium out of the cell. An outside impulse breaks down this potential and allows sodium to flow in, shooting a tiny electrical current down the axon, the neuron's transmission line. Sodium ions that enter the neuron are "pumped" out so that the transmission process can be resumed. Calcium acts differently. It appears to interact with certain molecules that compose the neural membrane, thus affecting its structural properties. Either way, such electrolyte actions could account for at least some aspects of disturbed behavior.

Recently, Ferris Pitts of Washington University produced acute anxiety attacks in a group of anxiety neurotics and in some normal volunteers with lactic acid, or lactate, the end product of blood sugar breakdown. It occurred to Pitts that many of the symptoms of anxiety neurosis resembled hypocalcemia, or low calcium in the blood. In tests Pitts showed that when lactate and calcium were given to anxiety neurotics the induced attacks were much milder. He concluded that lactate inactivates calcium and thus interferes with the transmission of nerve impulses. Pitts thinks his finding about high lactate and anxiety neurosis has diagnostic value, too. Today doctors have difficulty telling who is or is not an anxiety neurotic; a blood test for lactate could tell them.

Other studies have shown that a malfunction in sodium metabolism may also be at work in depressed patients, some of whom show retention of sodium during depression. After recovery, the sodium level recedes. Jack Durell, clinical director of the Psychiatric Institute of Washington, D.C., and his coworkers suggest in a current study that a genetic defect in the enzyme that serves as the sodium "pump" in neurons and other cells might produce abnormalities in electrochemical gradients in all tissues. "These might be so slight that the function of most tissues would not be impaired; in the central nervous system, however, they could result in the subtle change that predisposes to psychosis."

The third biological system is that of hormones produced by the pituitary, adrenal, and other glands. The pituitary and the adrenal compose an important stress-response mechanism. Under stress, the pituitary excretes a number of hormones into the bloodstream to help the body cope with the emergency. One hormone is adrenocorticotrophin, or ACTH. It stimulates the cortex, the rindlike covering of the adrenal glands located atop the kidney. The adrenal cortex releases cortisol, a steroid. The major breakdown products of cortisol are known as 17-OHCS (17-hydroxycorticosteroids).

Tracking down this important index of the body's stress-response mechanism, William E. Bunney, Jr., and his collaborators at the National Institute of Mental Health clarified the association between steroid output and depression. They found that daily levels of corticosteroids and depression in most patients went together—higher during acute depressive turmoil, lower during less severe depressive states. Most of the steroid changes *reflected* shifts in behavior, didn't precede them. Still, Bunney decided that the 17-OHCS level might give an early clue of suicide intent in depressed patients. Severely depressed people are often preoccupied with death and dying; the suicide rate among them is fifty times that in the general population. Suicides do not always clearly signal their intention beforehand, so Bunney hoped that high 17-OHCS levels would yield such a signal. Hospital records of a small number of depressed patients who subsequently committed suicide showed that they had significantly higher levels of steroids. The studies are continuing.

How exactly the three biological systems—noradrenaline, adrenal cortical hormones, and cellular electrolytes—interrelate physiologically is now becoming clear. First, noradrenaline has been shown to influence the metabolism of sodium. Second, evidence has come to light that the pituitary-adrenal function affects the metabolism of electrolytes at the level of the cell. Third, the steroid hormone cortisol influences some of the metabolic effects of noradrenaline. These few established relationships hint at the complexities that remain to be unraveled for a more unified biochemical understanding of depression. With such understanding will come new drugs to control depression.

Much more clear-cut are some recent findings about the genetics of mental illness. Kety and his associates are in the midst of what is probably the most ambitious research project ever undertaken in the field of schizophrenia. They are looking into the incidence of schizophrenia in adopted children of both schizophrenics and normal parents. The study, being conducted in Denmark, which maintains extensive personal records, confirms a previously suggested hereditary basis for schizophrenia. It had been shown earlier, for instance, that an identical twin is much more likely to become a schizophrenic if his twin is one than are fraternal twins or brothers and sisters in general. Kety and his team found that an adopted child who came from a schizophrenic family is much more likely to contract the disease. However interesting, this knowledge in its present form is not very helpful for prevention and treatment, but it could become so with additional work. Biochemical studies of discordant identical twins, for example, or of those where only one becomes a schizophrenic, could reasonably be expected to yield signs of biochemical anomalies. Knowledge of why such disturbances don't affect both twins could possibly lead to new medications.

Just how more precise identification of genetic factors might be achieved is illustrated by a brilliant finding about the genetics of the manic-depressive disease by George Winokur and his associates in the late 1960s at Washington University in Saint Louis. (Winokur has since moved to the University of Iowa.) This finding is the most specific indication so far of the genetic basis of any widespread mental disorder. The researchers studied 426 persons with mood disturbances, both manic-depressive and depressive. In this group they found 112 people in whose families mood disorders ran for at least two generations. Furthermore, they found a predominance of mania in the two-generation families. Some people with this condition feel elated about half the time and depressed the rest of the time. Mania is accompanied by hyperactivity, flight of ideas, meddlesomeness, and poor sleep. Others may have only manic episodes. Concentrating on these patients, Winokur and his team found that manic-depressive mothers had an equal number of similarly ill sons and daughters. In families where the father was manic-depressive, however, he was unlikely to have any manic-depressive sons, only daughters. This suggested to Winokur that a gene on the X chromosome, the female sex chromosome, was involved in transmission of mania.

To obtain incontrovertible evidence of this, Winokur and his team looked for and found a few families with color blindness among manic-depressives. The gene for color blindness (located on the X chromosome) was used by the Saint Louis scientists as a marker to demonstrate the link between the X chromosome and manic-depressive disease. They found that they could follow both the color-blindness gene and manic-depressive disease within a family. This wasn't a demonstration that color blindness causes mania or vice versa but a demonstration that, first, manic-depressive disease is a genetic trait, and that, second, the gene responsible for the manic-depressive state is located on the X chromosome. Such a transmission mode—through the female sex chromosome—can also explain why more women than men have mood disorders.

The finding is also significant in terms of diagnosis and treatment. From this knowledge psychiatrists could predict with reasonable accuracy which child in a family with a history of mania will get the disease later in life. Treatment could be more specific, since confusion about the person's disease would be largely eliminated. Today such confusion is possible because during depressive episodes a manic-depressive patient does not act or look any different from a person with depression alone. Mania is being treated today, experimentally and often successfully, with lithium carbonate, the long-term side effects of which are unknown.

Lithium has been a highly effective drug in treating *both* the "up" and "down" phases in manic-depressives. Although it may seem puzzling that the same drug could control opposing manifestations of mood disturbances, recent hints from animal studies suggest how this may be possible. Lithium has been shown to enhance the synthesis of serotonin in animal brains. Serotonin, in turn, apparently acts as a stabilizer of both "good" and "bad" moods, thus explaining lithium's two-in-one punch.

Even though the occurrence of manic-depressive disease appears to be almost totally genetically determined, the possibility of environmental effects acting on *all* manic-depressive cases cannot be excluded. One psychiatrist has described such influences as "environmental mobilization of a constitutional potential." Psychiatrists often cite tuberculosis as an example of such diseases; although most people carry the tubercular bacillus, only a few get TB.

Aside from genetic and biochemical defects, there is the possibility that damaged or convoluted anatomy of the brain causes mental disorders. Joshua Lederberg, Stanford University's Nobel Prize–winning molecular biologist, says he does not think that "biochemistry is the whole story. I think that there is a great deal of malfunction—I include development of the brain—that would be better expressed in terms of computer programming. If someone's perceptions are altered because of some misfunction in the hardware of the system, his software is going to get mixed up before long as well. And I'm not sure we'll ever easily disentangle this."

One big obstacle is the complexity of the brain. The brain really is one thousand organs, as one scientist says. Embedded in it are pleasure centers, pain centers, and many other relatively autonomous control and processing units. Unlike the liver, structured repetitively, each cubic millimeter of the brain is different. An incredible tangle of circuits and interconnections characterizes the central nervous system.

It's difficult enough to gain an insight into the structure of the brain and equally difficult to find out what's going on there on the level of the enzymes. Research on brain enzymes, the biochemistry of brain proteins, and on the structure of its interconnections is "not insignificant but small compared to the importance of the subject," says Lederberg. He notes that of the one hundred or so structural proteins present in the brain cells, each has a potential for polymorphism, or for occurring in several different forms. Just as sickle-cell hemoglobin, an abnormal protein in human red blood cells, impairs the blood's capacity to carry oxygen, so could any number of abnormal proteins influence the workings of the brain. In Lederberg's department a search is on for such abnormal proteins in the brains of mice.

Almost as little is known about the biochemistry of human and animal brain development. Yet there are indications that permanent biochemical changes take place in the brain during the critical periods of an organism's early life, the times known as imprinting periods. This is when learning patterns and the ability to respond to stress are established. It has been shown recently that a minute amount of the male sex hormone injected into a female baby rat determines the animal's future sexual behavior; the female starts behaving more like a male. A deficiency in another hormone, thyroxin, during a critical period of infancy means that the nerve cells in the brain do not develop normal arborization, the intricate branching that forms the basis for the axon's many interconnections. Such individuals show a severe deficiency in intellectual capacity.

The fact that a biochemical change persists in an organism is the basis of immunization. "It's very possible that the same type of response might take place in the brain," says Irwin Kopin of the National Institute of Mental Health. "Some proteins, some synapses are made when you are reminded of something—the biochemical memory is at a different level than the neurological memory, but some of the mechanisms which are used to induce changes may be similar."

Such changes may not show up even anatomically, yet the situation isn't hopeless where treatment is concerned. The alterations, whatever their cause, are still likely to be expressed in blood biochemistry. Lederberg explains that there would be no way to correct a defective protein per se.

> But if you knew just exactly the way in which it was malfunctioning, you certainly would be a step further.
>
> Take the sickle cell trait as an instance. We know that people who have 50 percent sickle cell hemoglobin in their blood would be stressed particularly if they got to high altitudes, because we can isolate that one function of the red blood cell where it's most vulnerable. Now if you could find that a structural change means that the organism is more susceptible to specific changes in ionic environment, or something of that kind, one could protect it. The schizophrenic brain is able to function under the same circumstances. If you can relate it to eventual deterioration, to the presence of some particular vulnerable protein, at the very least you could take some prophylactic measures. I don't feel that hopeless about it.

Hope, in fact, is the new keynote that the biological approach has brought to treatment of mental illness. And the work that has been done in the biochemistry of depression and mania is a great stride forward in a field where until just recently suppositions, even perhaps superstitions, prevailed.

CHAPTER FIVE

Stormy Weather: Fighting Rage

Hoping to rehabilitate such a violent individual through psychotherapy or education, or to improve his character by sending him to jail or by giving him love and understanding—all these methods are irrelevant and will not work. It is the malfunction itself that must be dealt with, and only if this fact is recognized is there any chance of changing his behavior.

—Neurosurgeons Vernon H. Mark and Frank R. Ervin
in their book *Violence and the Brain,*
describing criminals with brain damage

Assassinations, vicious muggings, and the high and rising U.S. murder rate have pushed the subject of violence to the forefront among American concerns. At times the nation appears to be oddly fascinated by the phenomenon. Consider, for example, the recent proliferation of grisly movies, some of which seem to glorify violence as a cult. We have heard abundant theories about the causes of violence, from permissiveness to drug addiction to racial frustrations—even to the legacy of the wild frontier.

Science is now venturing into this area of speculation and dispute, as a broad interdisciplinary effort gets under way to explore the biological nature and origins of violence. Biologists, biochemists, neurophysiologists, geneticists, and other natural scientists are probing with increasingly precise tools and techniques in a field where supposition and speculation have long prevailed. Their work is beginning to provide new clues to the complex ways in which the brain shapes violent behavior. It is also shedding new light on how environmental influences, by affecting the brain, can trigger violence. In time these insights and discoveries could lead to practical action that may inhibit violent acts, as, perhaps, a change in the way children are brought up, or treatment with antiviolence drugs. Such preventive steps might in the long run be more effective in controlling violent crime than either law and order or social reform.

Traditionally, the well-springs of violence have been placed either entirely inside man, as drives to be discharged, or entirely outside, as social influences. The reason for this dichotomy (nature versus nurture) is that until recently research into aggression and violence remained largely a preserve of either ethologists, observers of animal behavior in the wild, or psychologists, psychiatrists, and sociologists who knew or cared little about biology. Often relying more on literary skill than scientific soundness, ethologists have made some huge and questionable jumps from animal to man. They resurrected the ancient idea that man is inherently aggressive and that nothing much can be done to change his supposedly violent nature, an idea that dates back to Aristotle. Freud infused it with new life by equipping man with a destructive drive. The ethologists' ideas quickly caught on with the public, apparently because they offered an easy explanation as to why "civilized" man can commit atrocities. Such simple explanations also absolve society from doing anything very imaginative about violent behavior. The recent emphasis on law and order—more policemen, patrol cars, and other equipment—stems at least in part from these fallacious but widespread ideas or at least from the belief that violence cannot be suppressed fast enough by any other means. If it requires suppression by force, law and order hardly provides a long-range answer to how to diminish violence in a democratic society. Even short range, it has so far failed to make much of a dent in violent crime rates.

Sociologists and criminologists have stood at the other extreme. Largely discounting the biological underpinnings of aggression and violence, they have argued that violent crime is strictly a social phenomenon best dealt with by eliminating slums and urban crowding, by improving social justice, by spreading prosperity to the poor, or even by spreading the poor themselves, since they are prone to violence, among the more peaceful middle class, to "atomize" the subculture of violence. But programs in this area haven't been much more successful than the emphasis on law and order. Perhaps the rate of social improvement hasn't come fast enough. Whatever the reason, the rate of violent crimes has, curiously, been growing particularly rapidly even as social conditions have improved.

What conventional thinkers missed, it now seems clear, is that biology and environment are equally important. The human brain is shaped by experience just as surely as a sculptor shapes a chunk of clay. But the traditional mind–body dualism that pervades Western philosophy and the Judaeo-Christian ethic disregards the fact that the mind and body compose a closely integrated biological system. This dualism has deeply influenced some branches of science such as psychiatry.

Although the concept of the biological foundation of behavior is fairly new, it is already clear that influences on our brains are both internal, such as genetic and hormonal, and external, such as proper upbringing. What the new research shows, significantly, is that social practices such as child rearing leave their imprint on a developing brain. Improper upbringing can make a young animal, and probably a child, too, more susceptible to violent behavior as an adolescent or even an adult.

The brain is central to all behavior, and research is gradually laying bare the systems in the brain that initiate and control aggression and violence. Reflecting perhaps the evolutionary importance of aggression to self-preservation, the mechanisms that initiate aggressive acts lie in the most primitive and deepest part of the brain, the brain stem. The centers that control violence are situated in and near the immediate surrounding area called the limbic system. Here are a number of important substructures such as the hypothalamus, the focal point in the elaboration of aggressive and violent behavior. Destruction of the hypothalamus disrupts both spontaneous and induced aggression. The almond-shaped amygdala, located nearby, modulates the activity in the hypothalamus, whereas the septum, another nearby structure, seems to inhibit aggressive behavior that originates in both the hypothalamus and the amygdala. The cerebellum, in the back of the brain, and the hippocampus appear to be importantly involved, too.

All these systems are functionally and anatomically interrelated. Neuronal pathways speed along electrical signals that arise in response to sensory or internal cues (such as sight or thought) to activate or block the function of other neurons. Chemicals such as noradrenaline and dopamine, the now familiar neurotransmitters, ferry these electrical signals across tiny gaps between nerve cell endings, the synapses, to their final destination, where decisions are made. At the same time, the neurons are constantly bathed in background electrical activity that comes and goes much as do ocean waves. In still unknown ways, this background "music" apparently conveys information, too.

So complex is the organization and function of the brain that some of its estimated 10 billion neurons may have as many as 100,000 connections to adjoining cells. Decisions apparently are made much as they are in a democratic society: a neuron "votes" on the conflicting inputs it receives, then decides on proper action—whether to fire (transmit an electric impulse) or not. When an aggressive act escalates into a violent one, apparently more and more neurons are recruited, to create bigger pathways for the flow of pulses. Thus violence, as some scientists define it, is aggression gone awry.

Fortunately for the advance of knowledge about human aggression, the limbic systems of animals have recently been found to bear an amazing functional resemblance to those of man. So laboratory experiments with animals (notably monkeys, cats, and mice) underpin the still limited investigations of aggression systems in the human brain.

Using fine electrodes inserted into animal brains, researchers have induced a fascinating range of aggressive behavior. Cats that normally do not attack rats, for instance, will stalk and kill a rat when stimulated in a certain area of the hypothalamus. On the other hand, a cat stimulated in another nearby region of the hypothalamus may ignore an available rat and attack the experimenter instead. Destruction of the nucleus of the amygdala will turn a friendly cat into a raging beast that claws and bites without provocation, because the signals from the hypothalamus are no longer dampened by the amygdala.

Similarly, a tumor in the hypothalamus or the amygdala can turn a peaceful person into a violent one; luckily, such tumors occur infrequently. Surgically induced lesions also can increase or decrease hostile behavior, depending on their location. Corrective brain surgery on violent individuals remains highly controversial, however, mainly because surgeons lack precise knowledge of the aggression systems and know little about the risk of unwanted side effects from such operations.

Similar gaps in medical information inhibit manipulation of aggressive behavior with drugs that structurally mimic the neurotransmitter chemicals. Recent experiments by Peter Bradley, a British neuropharmacologist, show that a brain cell can be affected in different ways by the same neurotransmitter, depending on the state of the cell, the amount of neurotransmitter, and how often the chemical is administered. It also appears that during an aggressive act a general arousal of the physiological system occurs, of the same type as that which can be produced by such peaceful activities as jogging or even concentrated mental effort.

The complex anatomical and biochemical systems of the brain get their "orders" from the genes that determine behavior. Recent studies suggest that males have more brain cells that specialize in aggression than do females. This means that boys are more likely than girls to inherit aggressive tendencies. Very little is yet known, though, about the relationship between specific genetic defects and violence, how many such defects exist, and how frequently they might be inherited. Among the handful of anomalies discovered so far that some scientists have connected with violent behavior is the famous extra Y chromosome, which appears to be inherited by fewer than two men in a thousand. (X and Y are sex chromosomes: a normal male has an X and a Y, a normal woman two Xs.) The Y chromosome leaped from the quiet of the laboratory a few years ago and landed with a splash in newspaper headlines and courtrooms. The XYY males, usually tall, were said to have a natural propensity for violent crime. Some lawyers tried to gain reduced sentences or acquittal for their clients on the basis of their real or imagined extra Y chromosomes. In France at least one attorney succeeded.

Some imaginative work now in progress at the University of Connecticut suggests that the Y chromosome story isn't that simple. Researchers in the department of biobehavioral sciences, led by Benson E. Ginsburg, a noted geneticist, have designed animal-breeding techniques that allow them to "tease out," as Ginsburg puts it, the contributions of individual genes and chromosomes to behavior. Their findings strongly hint that an XYY male's tendency to aggressiveness depends on whether he inherited his extra Y chromosome from a peaceful or an aggressive father. The Y chromosome may act on the brain through the male sex hormones. Ginsburg and others are trying to find out how this process works.

Another type of genetic disturbance clarifies for the first time how aggression can originate at the level of the gene. Elevating genetic probing to new levels of precision, Ginsburg and his colleagues have pinpointed an interaction of two genetic anomalies in an inbred strain of mice known as DBA/1. In tandem, the two genetic irregularities make DBA mice, particularly males, more aggressive than similar mice with just one genetic defect. The DBA mice happen to be genetically susceptible to epileptic-type seizures that can be set off by a pure sound tone such as a buzzer, a bell, or even a jangling set of keys. The sound activates an enzyme system, controlled by a gene (as all enzymes are) and located in the brain region known as the hippocampus. In a mouse the network of neurons involved makes up an area the size of a pinpoint. The synthesis of the enzyme nucleoside triphosphatase, set off by sound, is not sufficient by itself to produce seizures, but it does generate tell-tale epilepticlike brain waves that can be recorded.

A second genetic anomaly operates in these mice and helps set off seizures. This system, unlike the first, is not sharply localized but is spread throughout much of the brain. It regulates the release of a chemical called GABA (gamma aminobutyric acid) that is believed to act as an inhibitor of electrical signals in the brain. The abnormality impairs the synthesis of GABA. The situation might be likened to setting off a firestorm in the brain and not having the water on hand to put it out. Or as Ginsburg puts it, with obvious poetic license: "You whip up an electrical storm in that region of the brain, and then you pour gasoline on it, light it with a match, and it goes whoosh!"

The same type of storm, and in the same spot, rages in the brains of certain people. They are either pathologically aggressive or have been made aggressive by stimulation of the hippocampus. This suggests, of course, that Ginsburg and his colleagues have found a genetic anomaly underlying aggression in both mice and men. In recent years, surgeons in some hospitals have stimulated different parts of the brain in cancer patients to find that area that might anaesthetize intractable pain. In a number of instances, where they electrically stimulated the hippocampus, they got the type of rage behavior that Ginsburg and his associates see in their mice. In one striking case, shortly after his hippocampus was electrically stimulated, a mild-mannered patient in his fifties suddenly brandished his bedpan as a weapon against the nurses and whoever else happened to be around. He later felt embarrassed and apologetic for his unusual behavior. In epileptics, those seizures can be set off even by flickering light.

The suggestion that the same genetic anomalies may be at work in mice and men is strengthened by the fact that the human brain has a GABA system, too, that apparently performs the same controlling, or braking, functions as it does in the brain of a mouse. And, interestingly, surgical lesions in the hippocampus that also set off rage reactions work only in mice that have a genetic defect in the GABA system.

The discovery of the consequences of these anomalies and of other types of brain damage shatters the assumption made by criminologists and sociologists that the vast majority of cases of violent behavior involve people with completely normal brains. Studies of criminals who have repeatedly committed violent offenses show that they have a higher incidence of brain damage than does the general population. Moreover, recent research is uncovering subtle forms of brain damage unrecognized until now. No one knows for sure how many people in the United States suffer from brain damage, but some doctors place the number at 10 to 20 million. Not all these are violent, of course, but in addition to them there are many thousands who suffer from delusions or other forms of mental disturbance that make them dangerous. David Hamburg, head of the psychiatry department at Stanford University Medical School, estimates that the nation harbors two hundred thousand potential presidential assassins. "Many manage their delusions on the fantasy level," says Hamburg. "Others engage in other forms of violent behavior."

What many people with brain abnormalities may have in common are pathways in the brain that failed to develop properly in infancy because of faulty upbringing, just as visual nerve pathways fail to develop properly in animals deprived of light. James W. Prescott, a young neurophysiologist at the U.S. National Institute of Child Health and Human Development, is the author of this seemingly daring idea that ties sensory deprivation in infancy to subsequent violent behavior. Prescott's theory of "somatosensory" (from the Greek for *body*) deprivation holds, basically, that pathways in the brain that develop in response to physical affection such as touching, cuddling, and being rocked and carried about do not grow in full when such stimulation is lacking. Consequently, the owners of such damaged systems behave abnormally. Prescott believes that the deprivation of bodily touching, contact, and movement are the basic causes of a number of emotional disturbances that include depressive and autistic behaviors, hyperactivity, sexual aberration, drug abuse, violence, and aggression.

This imaginative theory has a lot of factual support. For instance, a baby animal raised in complete isolation or a human infant growing up in a foundling home without proper emotional and physical care and handling both develop amazingly similar symptoms of abnormal behavior. They become withdrawn, hypersensitive to touch, and, at least in the case of animals, where such investigations obviously can be carried much further than in children, overly aggressive and even violent.

So pronounced is such behavior that the normal patterns of dominance among animals can be turned upside down. An especially vicious mouse raised by one researcher recently routed a mouse-eating snake when both were placed in the same cage. So aggressive are monkeys raised in isolation that scientists who work with them often pull the animals' incisor teeth to avoid being bitten, because some of these animals lash out at any moving object.

The somatosensory system includes two basic components. First, there are the nonmovement senses (somethesis), senses of the skin and of internal organs. Second are the movement senses (kinesthesis), with input from the muscles, tendons, joints, and the vestibular mechanism. The latter deals with whole-body movement in three-dimensional space, what a child or baby animal gets with rocking, swinging, and being carried about.

As Prescott explains it,

> Like any other sensory stimulus, somatosensory stimulation activates the sensory receptors—specific nuclei in the brain—and this produces biochemical and electrophysiological changes in the brain. The stimuli trigger signals through the sensory pathways in the other brain structures. These other brain structures—and there are many involved in the transmission of the sensory stimuli—pick them up, recognize them, provide interpretive meaning, and so on. These sensory brain regions have been mapped so that you can define very clearly the areas throughout the cortex that receive this kind of somatosensory inputs.
>
> We now know that the developing brain and the sensory system need stimulation for normal growth and development and function. Sensory stimulation is like a nutrient and if you don't get that stimulation during the formative years of brain development then that deprivation results in abnormalities and this is reflected in various ways. If the sensory deprivation is severe then you are going to get structural abnormalities, you're going to get abnormal cellular structures. You'll get two effects. One is what is called transneuronal agenesis—that is, a failure of brain cells to develop. And also you'll find that the cells that are already developed have been damaged. There are fewer connections from brain cell to brain cell. This is clear from studies of the visual system—cats and other animals reared in the dark are blind. There is no question that there is morphological damage due to sensory deprivation.

Prescott is suggesting that somatosensory deprivation—lack of mothering—renders dysfunctional certain brain structures such as the cerebellum, the "little brain" in the back of the head that controls balance and body movement and appears also to be involved in controlling emotions, such as pleasure. "With somatosensory deprivation you get a hyperexcitable, hyperreactive, and dysfunctional brain structure such as the cerebellum. It is sending out a mass of jumbled signals to other brain structures and this is going to make other brain structures dysfunctional."

Applied to Americans in general, Prescott's theory could explain at least in part the violent and aberrant behavior of children of both the poor and of those better off economically. Obviously, the two groups live in different social settings, which interact with the brain to influence behavior in different ways. In slums, where some criminologists feel that a subculture of violence determines adolescent behavior, improperly raised males engage in violent crime at ages as young as ten. In more affluent settings, equally affection-deprived youngsters seek a substitute for early deprivation in drugs. Drug abusers typically speak of their parents not caring about them. Research hints that this lack of early care may have damaged the youngsters' emotional circuitry. Brain-wave recordings of addicts suggest malfunction in the central physiological pathways that deal with pleasure. Perhaps not surprisingly, it's been recently found that marijuana seeks out the cerebellum in particular and settles there in strong concentrations.

Earlier investigators had observed how severe the effects of maternal-social deprivation can be. Rene Spitz, studying the effects of "hospitalism" on infants raised in a foundling home, found that such infants can die when proper emotional and physical care are lacking. Typically, a Chicago hospital boasted of never having lost a premature baby. They used to swaddle the babies and handle them a lot because the hospital had a large staff. With the advent of the insulating incubator, babies started dying. Life in an incubator singularly lacks activity and external stimulation for the infant. Many psychologists now realize that newborn infants are capable of perceiving and doing much more mentally than was traditionally believed. "If you put a newborn baby in a supine position in its cot and cover it with a blanket up to its neck all it does is cry and suck from time to time," says one scientist. "But if you watch a baby on the skin of its mother, without clothes but at a warm temperature, it shows a lot of things: rooting, crawling, grasping, and numerous anti-gravity postural responses."

The noted Harvard psychologist Jerome Bruner says: "We've begun to realize what a fantastic response capacity young infants have in the perceptual system. For instance, we find that four-month-old infants will suck on a pacifier in order to bring a moving picture into focus."

The early investigators (usually psychologists or psychiatrists) cared or knew little about the brain. So they described the adverse effects of hospitalism and maternal deprivation in terms of emotional, social, or learning deficiencies. To Prescott these descriptions sounded imprecise and disjointed. He knew that strikingly similar abnormal behaviors, including extremely violent behaviors, had been recently demonstrated in a great variety of young mammals, including rodents, cats, dogs, goats, sheep, and monkeys, when the animals were raised in isolation. Prescott suspected a common thread.

He knew that the senses (seeing, hearing, touching, tasting, smelling, and body movement) are an infant's only means of communicating with the outside world, which starts with his mother or a mother substitute. By studying the conditions of social and parental deprivation, Prescott was able to point to the somatosensory system as being the most important single factor in maternal or social deprivation. It appears to be even more important than vision. Lack of sight does not present an obstacle to normal development in either blind babies or blind monkeys brought up by their mothers. On the other hand, monkeys raised in single wire cages from which they could see, smell, and vocally communicate with other monkeys—but not touch them—show signs of somatosensory deprivation.

Prescott gleaned many of his ideas from Harry F. Harlow, the pioneering psychologist who did his work at the University of Wisconsin in the 1950s and 1960s. In a remarkable series of experiments Harlow dramatically demonstrated the effects of somatosensory deprivation on baby rhesus monkeys. Harlow placed an infant monkey into a cage with two surrogate mothers. One, covered with terry cloth and having bicycle reflectors for eyes, simulated the feel of a real rhesus mother but had no apparatus for feeding the infant. The other mother figure, made of chicken wire, was unattractive to touch but contained a baby's bottle from which the infant could drink milk. Harlow found that the infant clearly preferred to spend all its time with the nonfeeding mother substitute. Even when feeding from the chicken-wire mother, the infant would hold on to its favored terry-cloth version. Harlow concluded that in the affectional system of infant–mother love, holding and cuddling are more important than feeding.

Another outcome of this experiment was that female monkeys raised by the mother surrogate failed to develop maternal affection for their children. They could not, or would not, mother them. Like parents who abuse children, the monkey mothers would frequently attack, and sometimes even kill, their infants. In humans, too, researchers who traced back three generations the history of parents who batter and abuse their children found that the only common characteristic of such parents, regardless of social or economic class, was that they themselves had suffered from lack of mothering and affection. Harlow wryly concluded a recent paper:

Hell has no fury like a woman spurned,
With love not given, love is not returned.
The loveless female, human or macaque
In place of love will substitute attack.

Can such deprived, aggressive children—humans or monkeys—be restored to normalcy? Harlow's laboratory experiments indicate that rehabilitation is possible if done early enough. Young monkey mothers reared in isolation sometimes regain most of their normal maternal behavior when locked in a cage with their own babies. The infant clings to the mother so persistently, despite her efforts to push it away, that eventually the baby monkey begins to serve as a therapist. Similarly, some young male monkeys reared in isolation become less aggressive when forced to play with monkeys their own age or younger.

Among the strange aberrations in the behavior of both monkeys and human infants raised in isolation is persistent back-and-forth in-place rocking, as if the infants were trying to compensate for lack of such movement earlier in their lives. This is also a typical behavior pattern of autistic children, those self-absorbed children who do not relate to their environment. Anthony Ambrose, a British psychologist, has shown what such rocking by a mother or a mother substitute means to an infant. Knowing that crying often stops when a mother starts to rock a baby, Ambrose not long ago built and tested a baby-rocking machine. He then studied the effect of rhythmic up-and-down movement on normal babies only five days old. Ambrose found that, without exception, babies stopped crying as soon as the machine began rocking them at about sixty oscillations per minute, equivalent to a mother's slow walk. Ambrose concluded that inherent in the rocking movement is stimulation of the vestibular brain region that controls the body's movements in three-dimensional space. This region is located in the cerebellum.

The unusual importance of vestibular inputs was shown in another set of recent experiments. Going beyond Harlow's work, William Mason and Gershon Berkson of the Federal Delta Primate Research Center in Covington, Louisiana, reared infant monkeys on a swinging mother surrogate, a mechanized Clorox bottle wrapped in fur with a pie pan bolted to the bottom of the bottle. Their monkeys are much more normal than any of Harlow's monkeys raised with a stationary mother substitute.

Studying these monkeys, Robert Heath, a Tulane University brain researcher, concluded that touching and rolling around (muscle–joint–tendon stimulation) are the important sensory feed-in mechanisms. If one is deprived of these stimuli, the deprivation leads to behavioral deficiency in expression, an "imbalance between pleasure and pain," as Heath calls it.

Perhaps not surprisingly, Heath and a colleague, Barry Salzberg, have recorded abnormal spikes, or high peaks, in the brain waves emanating from heads of monkeys raised in isolation by Harlow. These changes in recordings, says Heath, are "very similar to those we have in psychotic patients and in violent, aggressive patients." Heath has also detected such deviations from normal in the EEGs of schizophrenics. In all these cases, the abnormal waves emanate from the pleasure centers of the brain. Heath's idea that psychoses of all origins are related to the diminution of perceived pleasure is supported by his work showing that pleasure receptors are located in the septal region and by clinical observations indicating that impairment of this region goes along with reduced awareness and impaired pain perception.

The EEG abnormalities in the monkeys raised by Harlow emanate from the deep cerebellar nuclei, from the septal region, and from the hippocampus. Because spiking—the repeated high peaks on the recording chart—in the cerebellum occurred at the same time as in the septal region and the hippocampus, Heath concluded that there is a direct connection between the cerebellum and both centers that deal with pleasure (which are in the septal region) and centers that deal with painful emotions, such as violence and rage. Interestingly, one of the latter centers, the hippocampus, is the same substructure where Ginsburg found that genetic anomaly in mice, which others have noted in disturbed individuals.

Heath now feels that "it's perfectly obvious that these sensations—muscle–joint–tendon stimulation, touch and vestibular stimulation which goes with changing one's position quickly and has to do with balance, must be tied in some way with the pleasure-pain system because otherwise kids wouldn't like the merry-go-round, where you are getting these shifts in position, or the roller coaster, or anything else that has to do with marked stimulation, or deep muscle massage and touching." To further corroborate the relationship between sensory stimulation and psychosis, Heath notes that a psychosis can be produced by shutting off the so-called proprioceptive system, which is responsible for the flow of signals to the brain that produce the sense of position of one's body parts. The proprioceptive system gives us our sense of balance but its influence extends to moods and emotions, too. "If you suspend a person in a tank of water, you get sensory isolation psychosis," Heath says. The New Orleans scientist feels that the cerebellar-septal interactions explain many other disturbances of mood and behavior. "We've discovered that the system responsible for hearing is tied into the proprioceptive system, so we're getting to a basis for the explanation of auditory hallucinations in psychotics. I think we can now see the physiological basis for these phenomena from two directions. If you impair the pleasure-alerting system you get disturbances in perception, and if you impair the proprioceptive inputs, you can get psychosis."

Further evidence of the cerebellum's role in violence comes from the work of A. J. Berman, a neurosurgeon at Mount Sinai Medical School and Jewish Hospital in Brooklyn. He has successfully modified autistic and aggressive behavior in isolation-reared monkeys by removing presumably abnormal sections of cerebellum that deal with the reception of sensory signals. In one experiment, Berman performed similar surgery on two monkeys called Ding and Dong, which had fought viciously and continuously. The operation turned Ding into a submissive animal, whereas Dong remained as aggressive as ever. Berman attributes the difference to the location of the surgery. Some tissue was removed from the midline section of Ding's cerebellum, but the excision on Dong was microscopically closer to the side of that brain structure.

Berman suggests that his findings may one day be relevant to treating humans. "Walk into the back wards of any mental institution," he says, "and you'll find children whose behavior is identical with that of Harlow's monkeys." The treatment most likely will be accomplished with very specific new drugs.

Many scientists now believe that an inverse relationship exists between pleasure seeking and aggressive behavior. For example, although touching and cuddling give a normal young organism pleasure, in a child or animal reared in isolation touching can trigger a violent attack, in dramatic contrast. A happy child or adult is much less likely to engage in aggressive acts than an unhappy one, for very good biochemical and neurophysiological reasons. Biochemically, anxious and agitated children suffer a deficit of serotonin in their blood and brain. Serotonin is a chemical mediator of the transmission of electrical signals in the brain. Neurophysiologically, as we have seen, there are systems in the brain that are anatomically linked and interact functionally. These systems often represent opposing emotions. For example, electrical stimulation of pleasure centers in the brains of men or animals eliminates feelings of rage. Electrochemical activity in one neural system actively suppresses an incompatible system that elaborates an opposing emotion.

In pathologically violent people the impulses resulting from somatosensory stimulation may not be reaching their destination in the brain. Pleasure is thus impaired or not experienced. This may explain, among other things, why rocking behavior persists in institutionalized children and monkeys reared in isolation. The children and grown-ups suffering from somatosensory deprivation may thus need additional neural impulses or neural energy. "This additional assist," says Prescott, "may be provided by the physical contact and 'excitement' associated with violent and aggressive acts." It is probably impossible to change such individuals by manipulating psychological or social influences. Neither jail nor understanding nor love is likely to help them, but correcting the basic brain malfunction may help.

"Although physical pleasure and physical violence seem worlds apart," says Prescott, "there seems to be a subtle and intimate connection between the two. Until the relationship between pleasure and violence is understood, violence will continue to escalate."

One way to deal with such malfunctions produced by careless child rearing would be to treat and teach potential parents. "American homes often are small institutions," says Prescott. "This is because mothers and fathers—regardless of class or economic conditions—do not appreciate, or understand, the importance of physical affection. Lack of it is the basic route to alienation, emotional disturbances, and violence and aggression in American society."

If anyone needed factual proof of that, he would have to look only at the backgrounds of violent criminals. Uniformly, these men were abused or battered as children. Assassins in particular have experienced a disruption or total absence of normal parent–child relationships. Says one researcher, "Love and acceptance are totally missing in their backgrounds."

Violent behavior can be set off by other environmental conditions. For instance, Leonard Berkowitz, a University of Wisconsin psychologist, showed that the mere presence of firearms can stimulate aggressive action. He tested groups of students, who were provoked and insulted by one of his colleagues. Later, the group had a chance to administer electric shocks to their tormentor. Students in a room where a gun was casually displayed gave the investigator about 25 percent more shocks than those in a room containing no weapons. The findings suggest to Berkowitz and others that easy access to lethal weapons (about 65 percent of homicides in the United States are committed with guns) not only facilitates the commission of crimes but creates an atmosphere in which violence is more likely to occur.

As in the laboratory, violence in real life often begets more violence. Marvin E. Wolfgang, a noted criminologist at the University of Pennsylvania, coined the term *subculture of violence* to describe the cluster of values, attitudes, and life-styles prominent among the poor living in slums. Violence in that setting is so common as a problem-solving mechanism, says Wolfgang, that there is no shortage of real-life models for the young to imitate.

Many other factors—frequently absent fathers, low income, unstable employment, poor living conditions—also bend the behavior of underprivileged youths toward violence, according to Wolfgang. Under all these pressures, plus in some cases a lack of physical affection at home, adolescent blacks have the highest homicide rate of any group in the United States. To complicate matters, adolescents undergo hormonal upheaval. Boys in particular become more aggressive as the amount of sex hormones in their bodies increases. Electron microscopy at Oxford University has recently begun to reveal structural differences between males and females in such control centers of aggression as the hypothalamus, for which sex hormones have a particular affinity.

Just how sex hormones act on the brain is unknown. They may affect the ease with which aggressive patterns are learned or make more rewarding patterns of action typical of aggressive encounters, such as large muscle movement.

With the aim of sorting out which boys are more vulnerable to becoming aggressively violent, David Hamburg and his associates at Stanford are setting up an unusual study program. It will see young chimpanzees, man's closest relatives, living in an outdoor facility at Stanford that combines features of the laboratory and the natural habitat. The six-acre enclosure will have an airportlike tower in the middle. The plan is to observe adolescent chimpanzees in groups and to follow their hormonal changes until they become adults. In captivity chimpanzees usually live to their mid-forties, and it takes them almost as long as man to grow up. Testosterone surges in a chimp about a hundredfold from childhood to adulthood, with a large part of the increase during adolescence. The aim is to relate these changes to changes in aggressiveness and later to follow up such relationships in man.

The still mysterious workings of hormones on the brain constitute only a small part of the enormous gap between what scientists have discovered and what remains to be learned about the physiology and biochemistry of violence. For example, says Benson Ginsburg, the University of Connecticut geneticist, scientists should find out whether men, through conscious control and training, can override the physiological changes involved in aggression much more effectively than, say, mice can. Another unknown is whether genetic instructions are so strong in some people as to mold their behavior completely. Answers to such questions could open the way to far more specific therapies. More effective antiviolence drugs, for instance, could be developed if we could delineate the particular enzymatic mechanisms in the brain that affect aggression.

Treatment with existing drugs, many scientists feel, is something like using a shotgun where a rifle is needed. Even so, some investigators propose that methadone-type clinics be set up to dispense drugs available now to persons prone to violence. Lithium might be useful because it appears to speed up the release of serotonin, a brain chemical that seems to inhibit aggression. Michael H. Sheard, a Yale neuropharmacologist, has had some success in modifying the behavior of violent prisoners with lithium.

Other novel approaches may emerge from studies that are under way. For example, development now in progress at Tulane of a vastly improved brain-wave recording machine would enable doctors to detect signals of trouble from deep in the brain without surgically implanting recording electrodes there. It may also become possible to treat damaged deep-nerve networks ultrasonically, thereby avoiding surgery.

To prevent brain damage that may lead to violence, some new tactics could be tried now. "Changing child-rearing practices is probably the most important single thing we can do as a society," notes Prescott. "We have to make sure that the children we have are wanted children." What's more, Prescott argues that the needs of an infant should be met immediately. Evidence assembled from different cultures does not support the view that such practices will spoil the infant, Prescott adds. "Contrary to Dr. Benjamin Spock," he says, "it is harmful for a baby to cry itself to sleep. By not answering an infant's needs immediately and consistently we not only teach a child distrust at a very basic emotional level but also establish patterns of neglect which harm the child's social and emotional health." Prescott also finds that discouraging breast feeding in favor of bottle feeding and separating healthy newborn babies from their mothers in modern hospitals are not advances but rather examples of harmful child-rearing practices.

Prescott and others also suggest that it might be a good idea to evaluate and treat children as early as age five if they show a tendency to brutalize other children or animals or have episodes of uncontrolled rage. Such youngsters, scientists say, are good candidates for violent behavior later.

Anthropologists have gained some intriguing clues about child rearing by studying peaceful societies. Prescott surveyed data from forty-nine primitive cultures and found in thirty-six of them an amazingly strong correlation between physical affection toward infants and lack of violence. In societies where infants were treated cruelly, violence prevailed. Robert Levy, an anthropologist at the University of California at San Diego who has studied tranquil Tahiti, found that parents on the island seldom punish children by hitting them. Thus, the children have no aggressive models to emulate.

Another deterrent to violence may be the practice of arguing it out. Societies that have developed highly elaborate ways of verbalizing violence are quite peaceful. In Tahiti and other Polynesian islands, people engage in "talking out acute anger, rather than taking physical action," says Levy. Similarly, Italians sometimes sound violent, but according to scientists who have studied Italy, there is a far lower incidence of violent offenses there than in the United States.

Nonviolence is not damaging to mental health, contrary to the beliefs of some Freudian psychiatrists. Furthermore, a society doesn't have to be backward or weak to be peaceful. One has only to look at Canada, England, Sweden, and Switzerland, to cite a few examples.

This nation leads the advanced industrialized countries in homicide and other violent crimes. Assaults in the United States occur nearly twice as often per capita as in England and Wales, and robberies are ten times as common. In 1976, the latest full year for which figures are available, 18,500 people in the United States were murdered. In England and Wales, West Germany, France, and Italy, which have a combined population about 3 percent larger than ours, there were only 1,900 murders, a rate almost ten times lower than that in the United States.

By contrast with the United States, these other industrial countries have more homogeneous populations, exert greater control over firearms, and operate with somewhat more rigid social structures. These differences may explain some, though not necessarily all, of the disparities in the rates of violence. In any case, it is clear that our methods of dealing with the problem have not proven particularly effective. Scientific investigation is at last beginning to provide surprising insights into why this is so. In time, the new research may lead to a much broader understanding of violent behavior and, eventually, to effective means of discouraging it.

CHAPTER SIX

How to Remember / How to Forget

Long term memory has to be chemical. How else could you possibly get memory from one part of the brain to another as indicated, for instance, by the Rapid Eye Movement (REM) research. These molecules may not themselves travel for re-storage, but they may in a sense "re-wire" the brain. Dreaming then may be what happens in the process, as the new memory molecules go out of where they have been stored during the day. This triggers old memories, which is what we experience as dreams. That's why dreams appear to relate, some 80% of them, to what happened during the day. Other findings indicate that if you prevent rapid eye movement during sleep, you have no memory.

—Dr. James V. McConnell,
professor of psychology,
University of Michigan

Dr. McConnell delighted a whole generation of journalists and laymen in the 1960s when he performed experiments with ordinary flatworms or planaria, which he had trained to crawl through a maze. He chopped up the trained worms and fed this "memory meal" to untrained planaria, which then seemed to acquire the memories of efficient mastery of the maze. McConnell called it "the first interanimal transfer of information."

As is the custom of "serious" science, it scoffed at McConnell's findings. We must remember, however, that establishment science has a poor record where acceptance of unusual findings is concerned, a trait all too typical of modern science, which has acquired some of the pomposity and other trappings of the medieval church. The French Academy of Science, for instance, in the late nineteenth century dismissed the existence of meteorites with the memorable statement that "stones can't fall from the sky."

Although he is an irrepressible optimist with a keen sense of humor,

McConnell gave up his planaria studies after bumping into the scientific version of the Nixonian "stonewall."

When we did our work with the planaria, it was too far out, too far ahead of its time to get the recognition it should have gotten. People refused to believe it. But now new work is coming along which brings us back into the world of recognition.

There is considerable evidence now that REM sleep* is "memory store time." During REM sleep, production of RNA and protein shoots up dramatically. In 1969 I hypothesized that the brain stores up memories during the day (maybe in the hippocampus) and "pumps" the chemicals out for long-term storage to the rest of the brain during dreaming. Little did I know at the time that Freud had said essentially the same thing 50 years earlier. More recently, this is something that researchers on the sleep mechanism have stumbled onto.

In lower forms, as with the planaria, we were able to indicate some transfer of learning, via the gut, via digestion. You can't do that in upper forms. In vertebrates, in mammals, digestion breaks down substances into component amino acids. Only in the chick is it possible to do memory transfer via the digestive system, and that only in the first 2 days of their lives, of hatching. In the higher organisms, the transfer must be done by injection via the blood stream.

Further support of McConnell's early findings comes from Georges Ungar's discovery of that mysterious "fear of the dark," or scotophobin, molecule extracted from the brains of rats trained to fear darkness. With that molecule Ungar and other scientists have been able to imprint a fear of darkness in various other animals (see Chapter 2). Still other proof of the chemical nature of memory comes from the recent discovery of the existence in the brain of small protein molecules, the neuropeptides that serve as codes designed to enhance or suppress memories.

Despite such tantalizing hints, the exact nature of the memory code

*Researchers divide sleep into four stages. Stage one is the beginning of slumber. Within a half hour or so of falling asleep, a normal adult passes through stages two, three, and four into deep sleep. The sleeper then reverts to the initial two stages until he enters a period of rapid eye movement, or REM, sleep, during which most dreaming takes place. The cycle of deep to REM sleep normally repeats itself three to five times a night.

remains to be deciphered, as is the actual location of memories in the brain. These are the great challenges facing today's neurophysiology.

Novel techniques are likely to lead to the breaking of the memory code and to locating its storage sites, however. In one such new project, Dr. Floyd Bloom, at the Salk Institute in La Jolla, California, has devised a clever system that measures changes in the components of a single neuron in a living rat as the animal is exposed to novel stimuli such as a red light.

Even without a complete understanding of what a memory comprises and where it is stored in the brain, however, scientists have been quietly taking giant strides toward restoring failing memories and bolstering normal memories with drugs or, conversely, helping people forget things they don't want to remember.

For instance, one big drug company late in 1977 was approaching the introduction of a drug called Lorazepam, which helps people forget unhappy experiences. Patients shown a one-dollar bill (the dollar bill is supposed to be one of the most potent visual stimuli there is) later received the drug and couldn't remember being shown the money or having experienced pain during particularly unpleasant diagnostic operations.

Other scientists have begun experiments on people with the aim of developing drugs that will help the elderly with failing memories remember things better. Some promising tests have already taken place at Northwestern University School of Medicine in Chicago.

The nature of memory has always fascinated us. Aristotle was interested in memory. In the late nineteenth century a number of scientists made important contributions to framing the concepts of memory. But serious study of the physiology of memory began only in the 1920s when the Harvard neurophysiologist Karl S. Lashley launched an ambitious search for what he called the engram, or memory trace. Lashley searched for the engram for thirty years. He trained thousands of rats to run mazes. Painstakingly, Lashley cut out pieces of their cortexes, hoping to eliminate memory of the learning. It was like chasing shadows: no matter where he cut, memory seemed to be a step ahead of his excision. Frustrated at the end of his busy life, Lashley wrote in

1950: "I sometimes feel, in reviewing the evidence on the localization of the memory trace, that the necessary conclusion is that learning just is not possible at all. Nevertheless, in spite of such evidence against it, learning does sometimes occur."

Running counter to Lashley's persistent belief in the engram were some disquieting facts about the apparently wide distribution of memory in the brain. Lashley himself found that damaging small areas in a rat's cortex merely blurred but didn't erase the animal's ability to execute previously learned tasks.

Surgeons operating on epileptics began to find some remarkable things about the persistence of memory in people, even after serious brain operations.

Wilder Penfield, a Canadian surgeon, pioneered in this field. Prior to excising diseased brain tissue, Penfield would stimulate the brain of the patient electrically in the region of the suspected pathology. This would help localize the spot responsible for the onset of seizures and would also call forth the type of experience that often precedes the seizures. Penfield and his associates found that they could produce recall of memories by stimulating the temporal lobes or their neighboring structures. That's a large area of the brain. Patients reported vivid memories of past events. When the electrode touched a spot in the brain of a young woman, for example, she exclaimed: "I hear voices. It is late at night, around a carnival somewhere—some sort of a traveling circus. I just saw lots of big wagons that they use to haul animals in."

"Oh, a familiar memory—in an office somewhere," said another female patient. "I could see the desk. I was there and someone was calling to me—a man leaning on a desk with a pencil in his hand."

Interestingly, even after a whole area surrounding the sites causing epileptic seizures is excised, no apparent memory loss occurs. This has led scientists to conclude that the impairment in memory comes about not because of the loss of a localized engram but rather because the mechanisms that code neural events so as to allow facile storage and retrieval of information are interfered with.

Additional evidence that the memory trace is not localized comes from studies of patients with "split brains," whose hemispheres have been surgically separated to relieve epileptic attacks. The left hemisphere has been shown to control language, with the right responsible for guiding artistic and spatial abilities. But despite the difference in the cognitive capacity between the hemispheres, there is no evidence of a loss of either verbal or nonverbal memories by either hemisphere. What this implies, of course, is that memory is spread throughout the brain.

There are obviously two different kinds of memory—short term and long term—and different mechanisms account for each. Investigations show that a rapid onset of amnesia is caused by drugs and treatments that modify the electrical conductance of the membrane of the neuron. On the other hand, drugs that inhibit synthesis of protein cause a slower onset of amnesia. These findings mean that electrical-chemical changes in the membrane that last only a short time represent short-term memory, whereas protein synthesis is responsible for the formation of long-term memories.

In seeking to tell what takes place during the fixation of short- and long-term memory, scientists have conducted some clever experiments.

In one such recent test researchers presented a shiny object to chickens again and again. The object was coated with methylanthranilate, a substance so distasteful to the chickens that they would shake their heads vigorously when they first pecked at the object. The scientists then injected saline, ovabain, or cycloheximide into the brains of different groups of chickens. The birds receiving saline showed little sign of forgetting the bad taste of the shiny object. Those that received cycloheximide forgot at a slow rate, with only half of the chickens pecking at the object an hour and a half after they received the drug. However, the chickens that received ovabain forgot the bad experience fairly rapidly, within an hour after training.

Ovabain is a digitalislike drug that has been used to treat heart failure. The scientists involved suggest that ovabain inhibited the function of the so-called sodium pump in the chicken's neurons. This sodium pump is set off by an electric impulse. Sodium is outside the cell, potassium inside. An electric potential in the membrane of the neuron keeps the two chemicals in equilibrium. But an impulse from the outside breaks down this potential and allows sodium to flow in, shooting a tiny electrical signal down the axon, the neuron's transmission line. Sodium ions are then pumped out so that the transmission process can be resumed. This process led Stanislaw Lem to remark: "All perception is but a change in the concentration of hydrogen ions on the surface of brain cells. Seeing me, you actually experience a disturbance in the sodium-potassium equilibrium across your neuron membranes."

On the other hand, the action of cycloheximide is explained differently. This drug inhibits protein synthesis. The fact that memory persisted during the early period after administration of the drug means to the researchers that the early phases of memory formation are not dependent on protein synthesis. "Ovabain and cycloheximide interfere with memory in different ways," they concluded. "We suggest that they do so at successive stages and that memory begins with a membrane store of limited time-span involving ionic metabolism and this is soon supplemented by a process dependent on synthesis of proteins which perhaps alter synaptic properties."

That learning brings about an increased synthesis of proteins and RNA has now been demonstrated in a wide range of experiments. In England, scientists found that an increase in those substances in the brains of chicks subjected to artificial imprinting, or letting a newborn chick follow a mother substitute, in this case simply a bright light.

For a number of years now at the University of Michigan Dr. Bernard Agranoff, a biochemist, has been erasing the memory of goldfish with an antibiotic, puromycin, which blocks the formation of protein. The fish are trained to swim to the other end of their tank whenever a light is turned on, to avoid an electric shock. The fish learn fast and normally remember the skill for a month.

But this memory can be erased, Dr. Agranoff found, if the antibiotic is injected into the brains of the fish within minutes after learning. Injected an hour later it doesn't affect the memory. Supporting the belief that short-term and long-term memories depend on different methods of fixation, giving the drug to the fish before the training does not affect their learning but does affect their long-term memory. Tested three days later, the fish have no memory of having learned the task. Drugs like puromycin are believed to act *not* specifically on memory formation but rather on the brain. In the process, the drug's action blocks the synthesis of protein needed for memory fixation.

It thus appears that membrane mechanisms are needed to start the long-term memory, but not for the fixation that takes place later.

The fact that in brain-damaged people long-term memory (as opposed to memories) is rarely erased except by the most drastic lesions has led some scientists to conclude that brain tissue—and perhaps all living matter—possesses an all-embracing ability to store information. Says one scientist, "After all, learning and memory have been demonstrated in animals made up of but a few cells and with no known nervous system." As another researcher puts it, "Brain evolution has not produced specialized structures that serve as general storage bins for memories." He expects, though, that these memory components might still be localized to particular nuclei and brain regions, at least in terms of information processing. Neurophysiologists are currently testing the idea that components of memory are likely to be found dispersed throughout the countless subdivisions of the brain.

The oldest concept of how memories are laid down permanently is that the brain simply grows a new structure. For a long time this idea was in disfavor because scientists saw no reason to believe that the mature brain continued to grow. For many years the notion reigned that once a brain reached adulthood, nothing changed. This gave rise to the picture of a static brain.

Soon, however, some imaginative research overturned that notion. In the 1950s, for instance, David Krech, Mark R. Rosenzweig, and Edward L. Bennett showed in experiments at the University of California's Berkeley campus that behaviorally bright rats displayed differences in the amounts of certain brain enzymes compared to dull animals.

Subsequently, the three scientists showed that rats raised in enriched environments, with a lot of toys in their cages, grew bigger, more chemically active brains than did rats kept in bare cages. Scientists had long recognized that a rich and stimulating environment early in life made a lot of difference to an animal's—and probably a child's—subsequent intellectual development. The Berkeley experiments provided the first link between an enriched environment and specific chemical and anatomical changes in the brain.

More recently, William Greenough of the University of Illinois showed that dendrites in the brains of rats trained to run a maze had grown more spines and more branches after the training. Greenough proved this dendrite growth to be a specific response to learning; he couldn't find such growth just by handling the animals.

All this work is bringing back into vogue the idea that growth can continue in an adult brain, with the brain incorporating new information. Obviously, dendrites cannot sprout in milliseconds, which suggests that memory storage begins perhaps with a chemical neurotransmitter that stores a memory for the short term, then instructs a dendrite to grow, if the brain decides to keep the information in long-term storage. Such selectivity in what to remember and what forget obviously holds an evolutionary advantage for any species. One has only to look at some known cases of people who can't forget. Life for them becomes a nightmare. Alexander Luria, a Soviet neuropsychologist, tells of a man with an apparently limitless memory. The man could memorize a table of fifty numbers in a few minutes—and recall it years later. His mind cluttered with trivia, the man's biggest problem was to learn how to forget the details he didn't want to remember.

In recent years, Gary Lynch, a young neurophysiologist at the University of California's Irvine Campus, showed that entirely new circuits of axons and dendrites can grow in the hippocampus of an adult rat.

The hippocampus is widely believed to direct memory storage. It is a relatively old brain structure that predates development of the associational cortex, the part of the brain that gives higher animals, particularly man, the ability to think. Lower vertebrates that possess a hippocampus but no cortex can learn through conditioning. But invertebrates that have no hippocampus are incapable of learning a conditioned response. The hippocampus is shaped like a miniature seahorse; hence its name, which means just that.

When a test animal learns a simple conditioned response to an auditory or tactile stimulus, a characteristic signal pattern flashes through the hippocampus. In effect, a picture of the animal's conditioned response appears in the hippocampus a split second before the movement occurs: the brain signal apparently forms a pattern for an ensuing muscle response. The hippocampus apparently decides whether such signals should be stored in permanent form, in new dendrites that are then ordered to grow.

The role of the hippocampus in laying down and retrieving long-term memories was dramatically illustrated in the case of one male patient, who has become known in medical literature as H. M. He is an American who had been operated on in 1953 to reduce epileptic seizures. Part of the hippocampus, which extends over both hemispheres of the brain, had been removed in some patients without damage to their memory. But because epileptic attacks appeared to involve all of H. M.'s brain, his hippocampus had been excised from both sides of the brain.

As a result of this operation, H. M. lost his ability to store long-term memories. He lives in a strange world where his newly acquired memories are limited to a few minutes. He was unable to recall events that occurred after the operation, once they escaped his immediate attention. Shortly after the operation, for instance, his mother, with whom he lived, moved to another house, but H. M. continued to go to the old address. He was able to mow the lawn but unable to remember where he had left the lawnmower. Day after day, he read the same newspapers and solved the same crossword puzzles. Each time he learned of the death of his uncle he became sad.

Although H. M. was able to work—he assembled cigarette lighters on cardboard frames—he couldn't tell anyone what he did unless asked while he was performing his duties. H. M. realized that he had experienced a memory loss and poignantly described his situation: "Every day is alone in itself, whatever enjoyment I've had, and whatever sorrow I've had. . . . Right now, I'm wondering, have I done or said anything amiss? You see, at this moment everything looks clear to me, but what happened just before? That's what worries me. It's like waking from a dream. I just don't remember."

From Lynch's research on the hippocampus there now emerges an entirely new, much more dynamic picture of the brain than anyone previously imagined. The brain is a far more dynamic, ever-changing organ than formerly believed—so different, in fact, that Lynch believes that the new concept of the brain is going to change ideas about thinking and about how the brain codes information.

Physiologists who dominated the thinking about the brain during the past thirty or forty years wanted it to look like a switchboard, a simple and comfortable way to look at this most complex of organs. It now appears, however, thanks to the work of Lynch and others, that the brain is constantly changing and remodeling itself physically, minute by minute.

Lynch and his associates have come up with a hypothesis that a second type of cells in the brain has a lot to do with this previously unsuspected activity. These are the glial cells. They are still widely ignored, and even the name suggests how little importance scientists have attached to these cells. The word *glia* stands for *glue,* suggesting that the glial cells are simply there to hold the brain together.

But Lynch's work hints that there's much more to the story. He points out, for instance, that though a human brain is nearly five times the size of that of a chimpanzee, there isn't really that much difference between the two brains in the number of neurons they contain. Man's brain contains 10 billion neurons, whereas a chimpanzee's has 7 billion. Our brains thus have only 30 percent more neurons than a chimp's.

Much of the intellectual gulf that separates man from chimp apparently results from the number and activity of those long-neglected glial cells. "We've shown," says Lynch, "that in the period before there is any axon sprouting, before any axon growth, the glial cells go crazy in terms of activity. The glial cells divide and they move through the intact tissue of the brain. They migrate through big sections of the brain to get to the active site. And the ones that are already there undergo incredible reactions. They send out branches that become very large. All this is going on before there is any axonal growth. None of these findings have been incorporated in textbooks yet."

Time-lapse photography shows the glial cells growing and shrinking constantly like amoebas. It appears that glial cells exchange chemical information and perhaps even impose directions on neurons, which is a far cry from their being an inert mass of glue. "It's a strange, bizarre system," marvels Lynch. "You know, the thought of these things crawling through your head, it gives you a different vision of the brain."

Lynch and his associates are trying to find out what signals the glial cells use to communicate with each other. With that kind of signal in hand, any kind of mood or memory could be controlled. "If you look at what is happening in cell biology today," says Lynch, "you can see that people are talking about chemicals being exchanged back and forth between the immune system, the hormonal system, and skin. In that sense, the brain may be no different from other organs, and events like memory and learning will reflect changes in its organization."

As for the memory code, one scientist, Karl H. Pribram, a neurophysiologist at Stanford University, feels that our memories are stored like holograms in our heads. A hologram represents the most sophisticated principle of information storage yet discovered. It is produced by recording the information in a scene with a laser beam on a photographic plate in the form of so-called diffraction patterns. These patterns, also known as interference, appear meaningless by themselves. But when illuminated by the sharp beam of a laser, the original image is reconstructed—in three dimensions. So far, holograms have been used mostly experimentally, but they hold the promise of three-dimensional movies and television—and commercials. Hologram advertisements could be "hung" in the air in front of stores for customers to walk through without apparent ill effects, except, perhaps, for some damage to their aesthetic sense.

Pribram suggests that both his own studies with cats and monkeys and the work of other researchers have shown striking similarities between memory and holograms. The similarity is based on the fact that holograms provide a complete three-dimensional image of the original scene. Several holograms can be superimposed on a single film plate and the images extracted independently when some of the conditions under which they were produced are repeated. The holographic film can be cut into fragments with each fragment, when illuminated, reproducing the entire image.

"These are properties shown by the brain's memory mechanisms that have puzzled scientists for years," Pribram says. In his work, Pribram found that although a portion of a laboratory animal's brain is removed, its memories can remain substantially unaltered. Physicists can perform a similar trick with holograms, snipping off a small corner and using it to reproject the entire three-dimensional picture. "Tear an ordinary photograph of your family in half, and half the family disappears," says Pribram. "Do this to a hologram and recognition remains unimpaired. These experiments bear out a common clinical observation. A man who has a stroke that destroys half or more of his visual system does not thereafter fail to recognize his family. The organization of the brain's memory store is such that particular memories are hard to wipe out." Storage of memory in a holographic form explains why long-term memory survives nearly all brain injuries. This would explain, too, our remarkable ability to recall a seemingly half-forgotten scene or sequence with the gentlest and most fragmentary of reminders: a whiff of perfume, a picture of a face, the mention of a name, a sentence that suddenly brings to mind a complete vignette from the past.

Similarly, a rat with 90 percent of its brain disconnected will still press a lever to stimulate the portion of its brain that remains intact. With only its brain stem intact, a rat can remember tasks it has learned for as long as six months, indicating that no part of the cortex or subcortex is absolutely essential for all types of memory or other intellectual activity. And the brain can store vastly more information than a hologram, which can pack 10 billion bits of information in one cubic centimeter of film.

"Distributed information and the incredibly large storage capacity —two properties of the brain mechanism in recognition—are thus accounted for by the model," says Pribram. He suggests on the basis of experimental evidence that the same set of equations and computations describes physical holography and image construction by the brain.

In a hologram, the individual traces are meaningless unless they serve as memories, with the peculiar property that the information stored cannot be immediately recognized as such because it is distributed over the entire extent of the image. That, of course, would account for scientists' inability to connect changes that occur in the content of neurons when learning is increased with anything that would even remotely resemble a straightforward memory code. The problem is that knowing how a transistor works does not tell us how TV pictures are made. Similarly, the holographic memory picture makes sense only when a laser shines on it.

Pribram accepts other scientists' findings about increased amounts of ribonucleic acid (RNA)* in the brains of animals following learning activity. But he feels that RNA plays only a subsidiary role in memory function. For instance, he suggests that RNA increases may merely reflect the synthesis of protein needed to establish new nerve cell connections.

"When the holographic model is taken seriously," Pribram concludes, "many paradoxes regarding brain function in perception become understandable. The outlines of the neural holographic processes are only now coming into focus, where not so long ago, only vague hobbits inhabited the land of neuromythology."

Even if it isn't entirely clear yet how memories are stored (the hologram model remains to be proved), it is becoming clearer how they can be restored. For a number of years now, scientists have demonstrated that memory can be improved—or blocked—in a wide variety of animals, from goldfish to monkeys. Serious work has also begun with human volunteers.

James L. McGaugh, of the department of psychobiology at the University of California's Irvine campus, has led the way in showing how animal learning abilities—and memory—can be boosted with drugs. Looking back at the rapidity with which tranquilizing and other mind- and mood-influencing drugs became available, McGaugh predicts that drugs and other treatments to enhance learning and memory

*RNA is the chemical that transcribes the inherited potential in DNA, or deoxyribonucleic acid. Interest in the relationship between RNA building blocks and memory soared when in the early 1960s aged human volunteers fed RNA rations displayed improved memories and sharpened alertness.

"are not likely to be ignored" by the public at large.

McGaugh points out that drugs have been used for many years as either real or imagined aids to learning.

> College students routinely use stimulants, including caffeine, theophylline (which is found in tea), and nicotine while studying. More potent stimulants such as strychnine and amphetamine are also sometimes used. Many of the stimulants are no doubt effective simply because they increase alertness and thus make it possible for students to spend long hours studying before examinations. If sleeping is the alternative to studying then stimulants can quite clearly help students learn. However, there is extensive evidence that increasing alertness may not be the only way that stimulants act to aid learning. Findings from studies using laboratory animals indicate that some of these commonly used stimulants may directly enhance learning and memory processes. Another stimulant, methylphenidate, is used extensively to treat "hyperactive" children. If the treatment is effective, then the treated child might well be expected to show improved learning simply because of an increased ability to sit still to listen, and attend. It might also be that methylphenidate directly influences learning processes, but this possibility has not as yet been studied extensively. In fact, little is known about the effects of drugs and other treatments on learning and memory in human subjects. Most of our knowledge of neurobiological influences on learning and memory is based on studies using laboratory animals such as mice, rats and monkeys.

McGaugh succeeded in improving memory consolidations in rats, using such stimulants as strychnine and amphetamines. (Although it's a poison in large doses, in small amounts strychnine acts as a stimulant.) He found that mice given strychnine learn to run mazes faster. McGaugh obtained similar results with metrazol, a convulsant drug, and with amphetamine. He even found that he could erase amnesia previously induced with electroshock by giving animals memory-enhancing drugs. Electroshock, it turned out, prevents new protein from being formed.

Lately, many scientists have become intrigued by the effects on memory of those mysterious neuropeptides that have been discovered to occur naturally in the brain. "My feeling right now," says Dr. McGaugh, "is that the main influences on memory formation are hormonal." He thinks that important hormones are synthesized in the brain as a consequence of electrical stimulation of laboratory animals. "We got the memory being made here in the brain, we stimulate the brain in that area and this causes these widespread hormonal influences which will either favor or disfavor the permanent storage of that recent experience. We feel that with neurohormones we're getting closer to the memory mechanism than we were with strychnine and other toxins."

In people, the stimulants of the hormonal "fixing" of memories could be external circumstances under which remembering takes place. Stress, for instance, is marked by increased production of ACTH (adrenocorticotropic hormone). In their outstanding experiments in the Netherlands, David de Wied and his associates found that the ability of rats to learn, which was impaired by partial removal of the pituitary, could be restored by giving the animals fragments of ACTH. This hormonal fragment thus appears to improve performance in response to stress. ACTH may alter the nerve pathways of learning along which new memories are then deposited. Somehow, ACTH appears to improve the ability of neurons to transmit information to one another, possibly by affecting the synapses, the connective sites between neurons.

Perhaps not surprisingly, the brain site most involved in the selective uptake of ACTH is the hippocampus. The reason for ACTH's affinity for the hippocampus may have been recently discovered by scientists at Irvine who showed that the first step in memory formation may occur in the hippocampus. This happened when they observed that characteristic signal pattern that flashes through the hippocampus when a test animal learns a simple conditioned response to an auditory or tactile stimulus. In effect, a picture of the animal's conditioned response appears in the hippocampus a split second before the response occurs. What's more, they found that a biochemical marking system accounts for the programming of memories into neural circuits of the hippocampus. They found a changing mosaic of strong and weak connections within the cell population, depending on the stimulus.

Research into the influences of the neuropeptides on memory consolidation and retrieval has turned into one of the most exciting and productive areas of neurophysiology. When the investigators' initial studies provided evidence of the neuropeptides' influence on learning and memory, their next step was to determine which aspect of memory was altered. *Memory,* of course, is a collective noun for a number of processes. Uncertainty still exists about the number and character of these processes. Scientists usually distinguish an imprint, or consolidation stage, and an output, or retrieval stage. They think that each stage consists of more than one process.

Assessing the effects of drugs on these time-dependent features of memory is turning into one of the most promising approaches in the study of how memory can be influenced by drugs. Pioneering in this area, David de Wied concluded that since ACTH fragments do not alleviate the physical malaise of animals whose pituitaries have been removed, the hormone fragments must exercise a specific behavioral effect directly on the brain. De Wied's discoveries inspired other researchers to try to find out whether the behavioral effect of ACTH is based on improved fixing, or consolidation of, memory. For example, McGaugh and his associates first trained thirsty rats to lick from a water spout, then administered mild foot shock to the animals while they were drinking. Small doses of ACTH were then injected into the animals. The scientists found that ACTH improved the rats' avoidance response to electric shock, suggesting that this neuropeptide improves the consolidation of memory. This possibility was further strengthened by the finding that the effectiveness of ACTH declined when the time between the training of the animals and the injection of the neuropeptide was increased. These findings about ACTH were confirmed by other scientists working with mice.

De Wied has suggested that ACTH and its analogues, rather than producing a general increase in motivation, enhance arousal in response to cues that motivate an organism. Several areas of the brain, including the thalamus, the hippocampus, and the septum, must remain intact for ACTH to exercise its effects on behavior. Electrophysiological studies support the notion that ACTH increases arousal. For instance, this neuropeptide elevates the excitability of the systems in the hippocampus that generates theta waves, underlining once again the key role of the hippocampus in memory consolidation. Moreover, the influence of the behaviorally active fragment of the ACTH molecule has been linked to rats' response to visual stimuli. This effect indicates that the neuropeptide portion of ACTH is far more specific in its activity than the changes in generalized arousal seen after treatment with amphetamine pep pills and other similar man-made drugs.

Arousal, motivation, excitability, vigilance, and selective attention are all used by researchers to describe the effects of the ACTH fragment. These observations have led investigators Henk Rigter and Henk Van Riezen of the Dutch drug firm Organon to conclude that the neuropeptide ACTH has at least a supportive role in memory processes. They also got indications from studies on amnesia that ACTH-like neuropeptides may facilitate memory retrieval, making it easier for animals to recall what they had learned. Amnesia can be induced in animals by exposing them to carbon dioxide gas. The animal loses consciousness, is revived, and is usually tested twenty-four hours later. The Dutch investigators found that amnesia in the animals could be reversed with the ACTH fragment.

One prominent feature of the Dutch research deals with the effects of neuropeptides on the performance of old animals. When the investigators first tested male rats 10 and 110 weeks old, respectively, they found no difference in their ability in learning to traverse a complex maze at the end of which they would find bits of food as a reward. But when they retested the rats three months later, the scientists found that the old rats had lost the maze habit, in contrast to the young animals, which had retained it. Dramatically, the researchers restored the old animals' ability to run the maze by giving them large injections of an ACTH analogue that is one thousand times more potent than the natural neuropeptides.

To evaluate the practical significance of this remarkable finding on people, scientists began to work with human volunteers. In one of the first studies, an American team led by Loye H. Miller found that the ACTH fragment retards the development of electroencephalographic signs of habituation to a reaction time task. The volunteers were presented with one of two different signals. One directed the subject to respond to a subsequent stimulus by pressing a lever; the other instructed the subjects to refrain from pressing it. In the beginning, the signals produced an expected E.E.G. arousal response, and the volunteers were allowed to get used to this response. Then the ACTH neuropeptide was administered to them. In the subsequent postdrug-session, the peptide-treated volunteers showed no habituation to the "go" signal but got accustomed, or habituated, normally to the "no go" indication. ACTH thus appeared to boost attention selectively.

In another trial by the same scientists, volunteers given the neuropeptide responded better to visual stimuli, but their recall of telephone numbers and solving of arithmetic and anagram problems was not improved, again supporting the observation that ACTH enhances attention selectively.

Attention is extremely important for short-term memory. For instance, when two separate speeches are played to a person through headphones, the listener will remember only the speech he has been asked to repeat immediately and apparently nothing of the speech coming into the unattended ear—except when the speaker's voice changes or the subject's name is called.

In additional trials, ACTH tended to improve maximum performance levels and to decrease errors, but it had no detectable result on short-term verbal memory. The important fact is that these effects were observed in *healthy* human volunteers, suggesting that anyone's memory can be improved.

How does ACTH work? De Wied and his collaborators suggest that the neuropeptide acts on membranes of specific target cells and, by inducing conformational changes, stimulates production of cyclic AMP, the "energy currency" of a cell. This in turn stimulates synthesis of protein, which allows the growth of new synaptic functions.

Another neurohormone from the brain, vasopressin, has been found by the Dutch investigators to have a longer-term effect (much longer than ACTH's) on memory consolidation and retrieval. They found, too, that vasopressin restores to normal the theta frequencies in the hippocampi of diabetic rats during REM sleep—and REM sleep has been implicated in memory consolidation. This same peptide also prevents amnesia in mice. The understandably excited Dutch investigators are now setting up tests on elderly people to see if their failing memories can be restored with the new chemical code words from the brain. It won't be long now before a true memory pill will be on the market. Most likely it will be based on those remarkable neuropeptides.

CHAPTER SEVEN

Blocking the "Death Hormone"

Genetically speaking, you've got a whole luxurious garden of mechanisms to make sure the animal dies on schedule. These mechanisms are control systems and the control system for killing an organism has to be located in the brain. Why? Because reproduction must occur before death. Otherwise you have no species.

—W. Donner Denckla, physiologist,
Beth Israel Hospital, Harvard
University Medical School

The idea that the brain, through its neurotransmitters and neurohormones—and possibly even through a life-limiting "death hormone"—acts as a clock for aging is a revolutionary concept. It is finally beginning to put some sense into a field long dominated by a lot of nonsense and pure charlatanism.

Until just a few years ago, research into the causes of aging offered such a confusing and fragmented picture that there seemed little hope of understanding this most universal of all afflictions, much less doing anything to counteract it. Armchair philosophers, introducing all sorts of misguided theories, held center stage in the aging arena. It seemed as though almost every prominent scientist, regardless of his field, felt obligated to concoct a theory of aging, especially as he got older himself. After World War II, Leo Szilard, a physicist, popularized radiation as a cause of aging, an idea since discarded. Leslie Orgel, a chemist studying the origins of life, came up with the "error catastrophe" hypothesis, in which a piling up of errors in the transcription of DNA in the cells eventually decayed the cells and the organism. This theory, too, has fallen by the wayside.

Some biologists sought to demonstrate (futilely, as it turned out) that a common mechanism caused aging in all living things from bacteria to man. This emphasis on the importance of the cell did a lot to boost consumption of vitamin E, which helps dispose of the cellular debris known as lipofuscin. But the debris, it turns out, is harmless, and this line of research unpromising. As a serious science, the whole field seemed stagnant. "Aging was such a fuzzy and poorly defined area," says Nathan W. Shock, director of the Baltimore research center of the new National Institute on Aging, "that young scientists traditionally avoided it like the plague. To recruit staff, you had to get down on your knees and practically sing 'Mammy' to them."

Now a dramatic turnaround is in the making, both in the quality of scientists in the field and in the significance of their findings. Revitalized by an influx of tough, imaginative young men and women unwilling to put up with threadbare speculation, research on aging is quietly coming up with some spectacular results so new they haven't yet hit newspaper headlines. The frontier has moved into the brain-endocrine and immune systems where, for the first time, scientists are beginning to see some coherent mechanisms of senescence.

What's more, scientists are beginning to manipulate these clocks of aging in laboratory animals, with the aim of resetting them to their youthful stability and thus prolonging the healthy middle years of life. The goal is to ameliorate disease in elderly people by slowing down the clocks.

As that becomes possible, the life-span intrinsic to the species will be stretched—for the first time in history. Man's built-in life-span has remained unchanged since the Biblical three score and ten, but a far greater proportion of people now live out that full life-span.

Progress in this new field of research has been remarkably rapid. In one startling experiment scientists recently succeeded not only in rejuvenating the disease-blocking immune system of old mice but have also extended the lives of the mice by one-third. The scientists predict that similar techniques will become applicable to people. The search is also on for drugs to prolong healthy lives, where, again, some promising medications are already in hand. A hunt is on, too, for aging hormones, the aim being to decipher their structure and to design antagonists to block their action. The state of research in aging has never been more promising. "A lot of labs, a lot of us," says Marguerite M. B. Kay, a young immunologist until recently at the Baltimore research center and now at the Veterans Administration Wadsworth Hospital Center in Los Angeles, "are on the verge of some very exciting developments."

This new work is being spurred on by the growing realization of just how urgent the medical problems of the aging are becoming. The number of Americans over sixty-five continues to grow—20 million today and expected to reach 30 million by the year 2000. In 1900 individual life expectancy stood at 46.2 years for American men and 48.3 for women; today it is 68.3 and 75.9 years, respectively. But this achievement, which raised the probability that an individual would live out his normal life-span, came mainly through the defeat of infectious diseases and brought a cruel by-product. For the survivors there lay in wait rheumatoid arthritis and the rest of Hamlet's "thousand natural shocks that flesh is heir to." Some argue that by prolonging lives medical science may have *increased* human suffering. Heart disease, stroke, and dreaded cancer came to the fore as killers of the elderly.

Researchers on aging are now becoming convinced that trying to pick off these newly important diseases of the elderly one by one is not the way to counteract them. At most, such a strategy might add ten more or less painful and decrepit years to an individual's life expectancy. The aim, rather, is to extend *healthy* life significantly, a goal that can be achieved only by defeating the diseases of old age en masse, by extending the longevity of the body's natural defense system against disease.

One leading researcher on aging, Roy L. Walford, a pathologist at the UCLA School of Medicine, argues that without quite realizing or acknowledging the fact the medical sciences have arrived at a crossroad. "Unless the basic rate of aging can be influenced," Walford wrote recently, "we are approaching the end of medical progress on a population basis, although of course not on an individual basis. There is less territory to win than formerly [in fighting the major diseases], and we must give increasing thought to the etiology and pathogenesis of the aging process itself."

Walford has prepared a "life-extension curve" to demonstrate his view of what the future holds when the breakthroughs he expects are made. This curve shows the young and the middle years greatly expanded. The last 10 percent of the survivors on this curve may still be senile, says Walford, but since the life-span will be longer, the percentage of senile persons in the population would decrease. "The popular nightmare of an increasing army of senile oldsters cannot be realized biologically," he declares.

As so often happens in scientific research, many of the most important new insights into the aging process have emerged as by-products of other investigations, as in this case with research into the nature of the brain. Until just recently, the brain had been largely left out of investigations on aging. Only in the past two decades or so have the intricate electrochemical controls by which the brain drives the organism begun to come into focus. The chemicals, known as neurotransmitters, including noradrenaline, dopamine, and serotonin, were found not only to ferry signals between neurons but also to control a whole range of emotions and activities from mood swings to muscle motion (see Chapter 1).

Where aging is concerned, the chemicals act through two adjoining parts of the brain: the thalamus, which controls muscle movements, and the hypothalamus, which governs the body's master gland, the pituitary (see Chapter 2). From the pituitary go forth hormones that control the processes of metabolism, growth, and reproduction. Other networks of neurons in the hypothalamus control hunger and satiety, body temperature, water balance, blood pressure, heart rate, and many other functions.

Some hormones, such as the growth hormone, for instance, act directly on cells of the body, instructing them to divide. Other hormones go to target organs such as the thyroid and cause release of still other hormones. Thyroid hormones in turn control the metabolic activities of nearly all cells of the body and are particularly crucial to the process of aging.

Hormonal activity declines with age or, more precisely, the response of the target cells to hormones declines, explaining why some organs lose cells. Until recently, one widespread view held that aging results from cellular and molecular changes intrinsic to each cell in the body, as though millions of tiny time bombs were ticking away everywhere in the body. "Aging in the test tube" or of cells in a culture was easier to study than the aging of whole organisms.

After observing an apparent inability of certain human cells cultivated in the laboratory to divide more than about fifty times, one scientist proposed that individual cells have their own built-in aging clocks. Strangely, he never mentioned that cells in the most important human organs (the brain, heart, and liver) never or almost never divide.

According to the latest findings, however, it's not the running down of individual aging clocks that causes aging in people. Those little timepieces, if they exist, seem simply to be cogs in the body's larger clockwork; or, as one scientist puts it, "The body is not a clock but a clock shop." With age DNA copying, or transcription (inside liver cells, for instance) slows down to one-tenth its youthful speed. But this speed can be restored to nine-tenths of its original value when hormones are administered, indicating that it's the hormonal milieu that acts as the governor of the aging process and not those tiny cell clocks running independently.

The cellular clock hypothesis also hinged on a clear demonstration of degenerative changes in cells' biochemistry. No convincing data of that kind has been forthcoming, however. Instead it has been shown, for instance, that DNA repair mechanisms in old cells are just as efficient as in young ones. Changes in cell structure that come with age *can* be seen with a microscope, of course. Those aging pigments called lipofuscins accumulate in old cells, for example, but there is no evidence that they cause defects in cell function or limit the lives of the cells.

Most intracellular components are continuously renewed, even in cells that last a lifetime without dividing, such as brain, heart, and muscle cells. "An old cell is very much like an old city," says one scientist. "While the town as a whole may go back many centuries, most of its buildings have been destroyed and reconstructed many times."

There is good reason why the life and death of a city is controlled by city hall, by the brain and not by peripheral tissue. If aging clocks were ticking away randomly in all parts of the body, the chances of an organism's dying before it reached puberty would be increased. Since nature is interested in perpetuating the species, it places growth and maturation, including puberty, under the brain's control. But after the age of reproduction is reached, nature treats an organism somewhat as a used-car owner treats his vehicle. "As long as you can drive the car back to the lot for a trade-in," says one scientist, "you don't care whether it falls apart the next day. The logic of evolution is the same."

The length of the "car's" life is under genetic direction. Identical twins usually have an almost identical life-span, whereas species differ sharply in their longevity, also demonstrating that genetic control sets the length of their life-span. Mice live about two years, elephants more than one hundred. But the mammalian species are amazingly similar in manifestations of physiological and pathological changes during development and aging. They all reach such milestones as puberty, maturity, and senescence in correspondingly matching fractions of their lives—strongly suggesting that the steps are programed. Many scientists now believe that the program for aging is encoded in the hypothalamus, perhaps in only three or four genes.

Two Soviet scientists have been particularly influential in focusing the attention of researchers on aging on the hypothalamus and pituitary. In 1971 Vladimir M. Dilman presented in the British science journal *Nature* a comprehensive theory holding that hypothalamic control of hormonal release gets out of kilter with age, leading to diseases. In Dilman's view, three main homeostatic, or regulatory, systems are affected: energy, reproduction, and adaptation systems. The disturbances in the internal environment of the organism and the efforts of those three systems to compensate for the imbalances lead to age-related diseases, Dilman suggests.

Expanding on Dilman's work, another Soviet scientist, V. V. Frolkis, in 1976 reported evidence that the hypothalamus undergoes structural and biochemical changes in aging. The rhythms of the bioelectric potentials in parts of the hypothalamus become retarded with age. The excitability of some structures in the hypothalamus rises while diminishing in other parts, Frolkis found. Because the hypothalamus is the brain's center for the regulation of metabolic processes, an aging and failing hypothalamus starts "misinforming" the body and diseases result. Frolkis urged scientists to start looking for changes in specific areas of the hypothalamus.

Young American scientists have now begun to do just that. At the University of Southern California's Andrus Gerontology Research Center, biochemist Caleb E. Finch and his associates recently undertook a study of brain metabolism in healthy aging male mice. Finch stresses the word *healthy* because in the past, it has now become clear, researchers often confused manifestations of disease with aging by studying animals that were sick, unknown to them. Judgments apparently were also made about human aging by looking at diseased tissue. For instance, the idea was widely broadcast that a massive loss of neurons occurs as we age. Newer research on healthy humans and animals disputes such generalities. The loss or damage (including senility) to brain cells is largely governed by disease. Similarly, Finch and his colleagues have found that loss of testosterone and shrinking of the testes occurs in sick old mice but not in healthy ones. The same appears true of old men.

Similar misconceptions appear to have been created about such other organs as the heart, kidney, liver, and so on. "A heart muscle is capable of going on for 200 years," says one investigator who studies aging hearts in men, rats, and dogs. "It's true that an old heart can't do as much when it's really pushed," he adds. "But in an ordinary resting state the old heart is just as good as the young heart—it just simply doesn't age." The older liver also seems as good as the young in disposing of alcohol, among other things. Finch says, "Many of the caricatured enfeeblements of aging in humans, such as intellectual decline or sexual impotence, are by no means as universal as the female menopause."

But if organs don't fail, what does? Finch thinks he has one answer. He and his associates are discovering that as the mice age, dramatic disturbances take place in their neurotransmitter metabolism. Particularly striking is the depletion of dopamine in the hypothalamus and the adjacent "pyramidal system," which controls the body's motor, or muscle, movements.

The deficiency of dopamine also accounts for the major chemical defect in Parkinson's disease, a movement-disorganizing malady. "We think," says Finch, "that Parkinson's disease represents an extreme development of what is a normal trend of aging—there is a general trend of impaired dopamine function in most mammals."

Furthermore, the dopamine depletion takes place in the basal ganglia part of the hypothalamus, just above the pituitary. It is this region, the so-called median eminence, that controls the releasing factors that trigger the flow of hormones from the adjoining pituitary (see Chapter 2). In a mouse this key part of the brain consists of about 100,000 neurons; in man it may contain 10 million. In either case it is a tiny segment of the brain, but these neurons may serve as pacemakers of aging for the rest of the body.

It isn't yet known what exactly happens to run down these clocks. Indications from Finch's lab are that the transporting of dopamine across the neuronal membranes is impaired. "One can begin to imagine a series of endocrine changes in which the brain has a role of controlling and at the same time reacting to the change," says Finch. "So there could be a kind of a cascade mechanism which results in disturbance of the equilibrium."

The cascade of events that Finch thinks is triggered by the age-related changes in brain neurotransmitters would include the turning on of various sets of genes by hormones. This could lead to disease.

In any event, one prominent scientist has shown that equilibrium can be restored. The late George C. Cotzias of the Memorial Sloan-Kettering Cancer Center in New York City first introduced L-dopa, a precursor (or a building block) of dopamine, as a treatment for Parkinson's disease. He fed mice diets containing various dosages of the drug. He and his coworkers found that animals on a heavy dosage (160 milligrams a day) experience a 10 percent gain in life-span beyond their normal limit of twenty-eight months. Many more of the mice stay healthy late in life. In contrast, a dose of four milligrams a day seems to have little effect.

Cotzias worked with a strain of albino mice that suffer from an unusual loss of brain cells. L-dopa apparently prevents a precocious imbalance of metabolism in their brains. The drug also imparts a marked effect on the pituitary, increasing its output of growth and other hormones and rejuvenating the mice.

In a day when the public expects miracles from medical science, results this dramatic might be expected to set off a run on L-dopa. But Cotzias was extremely cautious about extrapolating too much from his mouse studies, even though it is also known now that many sufferers from Parkinson's disease who take L-dopa are able to live out their normal life-spans.

The drug has drawbacks. Some patients being treated with L-dopa for Parkinson's disease have suffered disturbing symptoms of mental imbalance not unlike the signs of schizophrenia. "Right now," said Cotzias in a 1977 interview, "L-dopa, being the very powerful drug it is, should be sold only for medical purposes intended, and nothing else."

Pharmaceutical companies have come up with variants that don't have such side effects. And food faddists will be pleased to learn that their old favorite, wheat germ, is one source of L-dopa. The velvet bean, once grown in the South for fodder, is an even richer source. At this point it's not known for certain whether such foods can even influence dopamine levels in the brain, much less whether they could affect aging (see Chapter 3).

The depletion of dopamine and a slowdown in adrenaline turnover are also implicated now in the onset of menopause in women. No other alteration that comes with age is more clearly defined as being mediated by hormones as the female change of life. Clearly not related to any disease condition, menopause represents a programed event that, it is now clear, is controlled by the brain.

Menopause is marked by the failure of the ovaries to produce estrogen. It was thought until recently that it was caused by the loss of oocytes, or egg cells, from the ovary. But ovaries of postmenopausal women were found to contain an average of 10,900 oocytes, each a potential baby.

It is clear now that changes in the hypothalamus, not the ovaries, are responsible for the onset of menopause. Old ovaries transplanted into young rats begin to function, whereas young ovaries placed into an old animal do not. High levels of both dopamine and adrenaline appear to be needed for the cyclic discharge of pituitary hormones that drive the ovarian cycles.

In a fascinating series of experiments that are a follow-up on Finch's work, Joseph Meites and colleagues at Michigan State University have restarted estrous cycles, or reproductive "heat," in old rats by stimulating the animals' hypothalamic regions electrically, as well as by administering neurotransmitter chemicals and L-dopa. The Michigan scientists found that a functional deterioration occurs in the aging hypothalamus and pituitary, a decline that leads to poorer release of gonadotropins, which influence ovulation.

It also appears that the successful route to treatment of breast cancer may be through the brain. In 1971 Meites and his coworkers reported that L-dopa given to rats helped reduce the incidence of mammary cancers. By boosting dopamine levels in the hypothalamus, L-dopa apparently decreased the amount of prolactin in the blood (increased prolactin output in women and rats can lead to breast cancer). Doctors are now beginning to use L-dopa to treat women with breast cancer as a result of that work with animals. These experimental treatments are so new that it isn't known yet whether L-dopa can be used preventively.

Drugs to retard aging are also being sought in an intriguing project at the University of California at Berkeley. Narrowing down the mechanisms of aging, physiologists Paola S. Timiras and Paul E. Segall have been feeding laboratory rats a diet deficient in tryptophan, an essential amino acid. Tryptophan is needed not only for normal protein synthesis but also because it is the precursor of the neurotransmitter serotonin. (L-dopa, in contrast, is known to lower brain serotonin levels while it boosts the dopamine content.)

The Berkeley experiment is a refinement of the famous work by Cornell biologist Clive McCay who in 1939 succeeded in extending the lives of rats by 40 percent by feeding them a diet low in fats and sugar. McCay's rats seemed to undergo slowed development, and the diseases of old age were postponed in the animals. Until now, McCay's experiments have stood as the landmark work in the prolongation of animal life.

The California scientists are employing tryptophan as a specific tool to pinpoint the centers in the hypothalamus responsible for aging. Diets low in tryptophan had been successfully employed to delay growth and maturation in the chick, and Timiras and Segall have significantly extended that work. They have shown that rats can be maintained in an immature state for nearly two years. Even that may not be the limit; it's simply how long they have observed the rats so far.

Surprisingly, when put back on normal diets the tiny tryptophan-deficient animals suddenly undergo tremendous rejuvenation as their growth spurts back toward normal. Females long past reproductive age bear litters; these rats are capable of reproducing at ages of up to twenty-eight months, when nearly half the control animals (which are infertile at seventeen months) are dead. The rejuvenated rats have a better than equal chance of surviving past thirty months, showing a slight increase in average life-span.

These rats don't live longer, says Segall, because it seems that the longer the period of deprivation the more rapid the demise of the rat as it enters senescence. In other words, rats put back on a normal diet seem to restart a timing mechanism in the brain. Segall thinks that important clues to the aging process are hidden in that transition.

The link between neurotransmission and neuroendocrine function also comes into focus in the Timiras-Segall experiments. Body growth, reproductive activity, and coat appearance of the animals all depend on hormones. During undernutrition, the pituitary produces many of the hormones at such a reduced level that long-term underfeeding has been compared to surgical or chemical removal of the gland. Catch-up growth and extended reproductive capabilities after returning to a normal diet suggest a recovery in pituitary function.

Some of the effects of undernutrition on people seem similar to those produced in rats. In women, long-term undernourishment causes an inability to conceive. When people return to a normal diet, a marked oscillation in steroid hormone level follows. This pattern resembles the hormonal uncertainties of adolescence before complete maturation of the brain imposes firm control on the hypothalamic–pituitary axis.

Most Americans, of course, have to worry not about undernourishment but overeating. One specialist in obesity raises the intriguing question of whether the overfeeding of American youths might not lead to their faster aging and a shorter life-span. As American children overeat, they reach puberty sooner and grow bigger than their predecessors, yet the relation of prepuberty to the total life-span appears pretty definitely set in most mammals. In other words, earlier puberty may lead to shorter life.

Although no one has yet deliberately tried on humans a counterpart of the McCay low-calorie rat diet, the diets of long-lived mountaineers in the Caucasus, Ecuador, and Hunza tend to resemble the McCay rat diet more closely than they do the National Academy of Sciences' recommended daily consumption of twenty-six hundred calories for a moderately active person. The diet of the Ecuadorians typically is only seventeen hundred calories. Vilcabamba, the village where these people are concentrated, boasts among its eight hundred residents nine who are more than one hundred years old. Nearly all the elderly Ecuadorians work in the fields, also supporting recent findings about mice at the Jackson Laboratory in Bar Harbor, Maine. Research there shows that the longest-lived mice are the ones that are kept slightly underfed and given a new learning task every day. Perhaps not surprisingly, scientists have also noticed that the menopause in Ecuadorian women sets in about five years later than in American women, suggesting a slowed-down aging clock. Segall thinks that a combination of a life-prolonging diet and drugs will eventually emerge from the current research.

Long before Segall or anyone else develops an antiaging pill, improvements in the health of the elderly are likely to come from another direction, from bolstering the immune system. "If we could reconstitute the immune system perfectly," says Walford of UCLA, "I think people could live another fifty years."

The body's guardian against disease, the immune system consists mainly of lymphocytes, or white blood cells generated by stem cells in the bone marrow. Some stem cells migrate to the thymus, a gland high under the breastbone, and develop into T (for thymus) lymphocytes, or T cells. From the thymus the T cells enter the blood and the lymphoid tissue. There they are the killer cells that attack cancer cells, as well as viruses, bacteria, fungi, and other invaders of the body.

Some other stem cells from the bone marrow move directly to the peripheral lymphoid tissue and become B (for bone marrow) lymphocytes, or B cells. They produce antibody molecules that lock on to invading foreign objects and incapacitate them. To be really efficient, however, B cells must be stimulated in some still unknown way by the T cells. The debris of the battles against invaders is cleared by macrophages, cells that act as microscopic garbage trucks.

Many studies now implicate the thymus as a key clock in the aging of the immune system. Not many years ago, scientists didn't even know what role the thymus played in the body, but it was generally thought to have something to do with sexual maturation. The presumed connection suggested itself because the thymus starts shrinking in size quite early in life, even before puberty. There appears to be a link between the hypothalamus, the pituitary, and the thymus. In any event, the slow atrophy of the thymus is paralleled by a decrease in the number of T cells.

As a result, older people become more susceptible to a whole range of diseases, from cancer to diabetes. Even heart disease is beginning to be viewed now as the result of a decline in the efficiency of the immune system. Atherosclerosis, the major form of the hardening of the arteries, appears to be caused by patches of living tissue not dividing properly on arterial walls, a process similar to cancer. (Cholesterol, the old bugaboo in heart disease, may play a secondary role as a carrier of chemicals damaging to arterial cells.)

Simultaneously, in aging the autoimmune response, in which lymphocytes mistakenly attack the body's own cells as foreign, goes up, bringing with it such autoimmune diseases as rheumatoid arthritis.

This decline is retarded in undernourished mice, rats, and fish. When McCay extended the lives of rats in the mid-1930s by underfeeding them, he noted that the incidence of cancer and other diseases of old age was postponed in his rodents. McCay didn't look specifically at the immune system of the rats. There wasn't much he could have seen in those days. So recent are the advances in immunology that only in the 1950s were the lymphocytes unequivocally identified as being responsible for immune reactions. And it wasn't until the 1960s that the lymphocytes were separated into the two distinct functional classes.

Immunologists who have entered the field of research on aging in recent years not only have dissected the decline of the immune response with sophisticated new techniques but have already started trying to correct the defects. We'll soon be hearing a new term, *immunoengineering.* With certain drugs, scientists have partially restored the immune systems of laboratory animals.

In 1975 came what looks like a big break. Takashi Makinodan and associates at the National Institute of Aging's Baltimore center succeeded in transplanting both thymuses from young mice as well as bone marrow into older animals. Because genetically inbred strains of mice are used, there are no rejection problems in such transplants. Newly equipped with both components of the immune system, the mice apparently started making antibodies against invading bacteria and viruses. Immune systems of nineteen-month-old mice were rejuvenated to the level of four-month-old control animals. In human terms, this would be like imparting the functions of a twenty-year-old's immune system to a sixty-year-old man.

Superimposed on these experiments came an unplanned additional one when a Sendai virus, the mouse equivalent of influenza, raced through the nine-thousand-mouse colony at the center. Interestingly, Makinodan's mice with the enhanced immune systems survived, though some of the unprotected old mice used as controls died. Most of the mice with the enhanced immune system lived about one third beyond their normal life-span.

The scientists are understandably excited by the progress so far. "We can trip the clock," exclaims Marguerite Kay, who works with Makinodan. "We can make mice live longer."

Success with bone-marrow transplants in children to ameliorate inherited blood disorders, leukemia, and other conditions hints at the possibility of applying the technique to older people, too. At least a dozen medical teams in the United States are doing bone-marrow transplants (injections of cells into a recipient's veins with a hypodermic needle), and some patients are still alive almost six years after the transplants.

Makinodan has also taken lymphocytes from mice and preserved them in a frozen state for months. Later, after thawing the cells, he successfully put them back into the aged animals. He thinks that the technique may be applied to revitalize the immune systems of old people. The cells would be taken from a person's bloodstream while he is a teen-ager for use later in life.

A slight lowering of the body's temperature may be still another way of extending the healthy life-span. Walford of UCLA has doubled and tripled the lives of annual fish (a kind of tropical fish that normally live one year) by keeping them at lower than normal temperatures. Now he plans to extend such experiments to mice. Walford has spent some time in India, studying yogis, who can control their body temperatures to some extent. He hopes to train mice to drop their temperatures on command. Repeated shocks to the animals at the peak of the temperature curve should force them to keep their bodies cooler than normal, Walford thinks. A mouse would have a tiny transmitter-thermometer in its abdomen that would broadcast the animal's temperature to recording instruments.

Animals that hibernate seem to live longer. Bats, which spend part of their lives hibernating, are around for fourteen years, similarly sized rats for only three. Whether temperature lowering can be safely applied to man isn't yet known. Walford thinks it can. "Our body temperature is set by evolutionary pressure probably at an optimal level for doing physical labor," he says. "Most of us aren't doing heavy physical labor anymore."

But the most spectacular approach to extending the healthy years of life is being pursued by W. Donner Denckla of Beth Israel Hospital at Harvard Medical School. A Harvard-trained physiologist, Denckla thinks that a specific "death hormone" released by the pituitary after puberty starts the clock of aging running.

"The mechanism for killing an organism must be tied in with puberty," says Denckla. "If it weren't, you'd throw out the baby with the bathwater." That is, reproduction must obviously precede death for any species to survive.

The onset of reproduction is controlled by the hypothalamus in the brain, and the mechanism for killing an organism, Denckla argues, must be connected with it. We know that the pituitary is supervised by the hypothalamus. "For safety's sake," says Denckla, "you must have the same biological clock that drives reproduction drive the mechanism for death—with a lag of about 10 years."

He points out that when man lived in the wild, most people died at about the age of twenty-five. Many women died in childbirth, and twenty-five-year-old men would lose out in competition with younger men, whom they couldn't outrun and beat up, or would be killed by stronger animals. Denckla thinks it's no accident that men reach the peak of their physical strength at nineteen. He sees that as support for his belief that man has always had a built-in mechanism of death, "like a pyromaniac putting his house on fire." What has happened in the course of evolution, Denckla says, is that the same mechanism that caused man's demise at twenty-five now kills him at seventy—which is the natural life-span. Adds Denckla, "The death mechanism started at 10, even in the wild."

There are remarkable examples in nature of precisely programed death mechanisms operated by hormones. In a species of Australian mole the male reaches sexual maturity at one year of age and dies dramatically after copulation. The cause of death is massive hormonal flooding. The female mole lives on to three years. Similarly, Pacific Northwest salmon go from youthful vigor to senile weakness and death in barely two weeks after reaching their spawning grounds and depositing their eggs. A flood of pituitary hormones kills the fish. (But taking out the pituitary stops the salmon from dying after spawning.) Denckla became convinced that a similar process takes place in man over several decades. "To quote Eliot," he says, "man dies 'not with a bang but with a whimper.' "

Denckla's theory is about not aging but death, a subject most other researchers on aging don't even consider separately. Most conventional researchers view aging as a deterioration that sets in with time. But Denckla argues that aging means simply that an observable change takes place with time, without telling us whether the change is good or bad.

> I'm not interested in aging. I'm only interested in death. That is a vector which has a direction. Aging has no definable vector, either good or bad.
>
> When you start talking about death, you are no longer without any clear landmarks because now you can talk about diseases. When is man healthiest? As a 10-year-old boy or girl. So the process of dying doesn't start at 50; it starts at 11. The first mistake aging researchers make is not to take that into account. Ninety percent of the research is done on older animals which are compared with still older animals, when most of the damage is already done. And then they try to build up the big differences. There aren't any. They can't find any because their frame of reference is wrong. If you look at death, aging starts at puberty. So now you begin to get into a better frame of reference.

The other difference between Denckla and armchair theorists on aging is that Denckla has observed and investigated firsthand the causes of death in man. As a young intern he was startled to discover that people didn't die of the six or seven hundred alleged causes but only of the two major ones: failure of the heart or of the immune system (if cancer is considered a failure of immune surveillance, as it now is by many specialists).

There are, of course, genetic diseases such as hemophilia, Huntington's chorea, and late-onset diabetes. They account for about 6 to 10 percent of total deaths. The biggest killers are cardiovascular disease with 50 percent; cancer with 30 percent, and infection, about 14 percent.

As Denckla notes further:

> There are only two systems in the body that cause death. This isn't in any medical text because nobody has bothered with that. Because that's not what medical people are interested in. They are interested in diseases which occurred five minutes, or five days before death. Aging theoreticians don't even know about the diseases. But I'm desperately interested in the diseases because that's what causes death. The diseases themselves are not like a nail or a piece

of gravel that cause accidents by blowing out a car's tire—it's the 40,000 miles of previous wear that went into it. So, what I'm saying is let's go back and find the absolute irreducible minimum number of systems in the body that fail with age. There are only two. Now you've got something scientifically that you can deal with.

When he became a research scientist, Denckla began to study thyroid hormones because the thyroid gland controls the competence of both systems. Both fail in people with hypothyroidism, or thyroid deficiency.

In the early 1970s Denckla was startled to discover that although levels of thyroid remained almost unchanged in old rats, the responsiveness of their tissues to thyroxin declined to about one-third its youthful value.

Denckla had a historical precedent of intense scientific interest in the thyroid and aging. At the beginning of this century, a flurry of excitement accompanied the finding that there seemed to be similarities between symptoms of normal old age and hypothyroidism in young people. However, these early investigators didn't know what Denckla would know in the 1970s, that no matter how much thyroid they gave old people, they could not rejuvenate them, because the responsiveness of their tissues to thyroid hormones had declined dramatically. Simply measuring the level of thyroid hormones in the body gave no clue to that startling fact, because the thyroid levels remained the same in young and old.

Unfortunately for those early experimenters, however, there was—and is—one type of cell in the body that responds to higher doses of thyroid hormones all too well, regardless of a person's age. These cells make up the sinus node, the apparatus that controls the heart rate. Not surprisingly, when those early investigators significantly raised the thyroid dose, a number of their patients instead of being rejuvenated died of heart failure. Since thyroid replacement therapy didn't work (or so it seemed on the surface), those early experimenters gave up the work.

They could not have gone much further in those days because only now is the molecular basis for the slow decline in tissue sensitivity being revealed. In the past year or so, scientists in different laboratories established that thyroid receptors on cell membranes in the brain and in various parts of the body decrease with age in their numbers. These receptors float in the membranes like ships at sea, allowing a hormone molecule to dock with them. The molecule then either sends a signal to the cell's nucleus or even enters the cell directly, depending on the nature of the cell, and influences the cell's metabolic activity by commanding the DNA in its nucleus to proceed with cell division or some other desired action.

Because the thyroid hormones are so centrally involved in metabolic processes, their lessened action would lead to deterioration of cell activity and eventually to disease.

The thyroid gland controls maximum strength and psychomotor reaction time in man, the ability to "run fast" in all kinds of ways. If a woman's thyroid gland is surgically removed, the woman stops ovulating. In fact, the most common form of sterility, produced by hypothyroidism, is easily curable with thyroid hormones.

Denckla thinks it's the "death hormone" that starts flowing from the pituitary shortly after puberty that causes the deterioration in tissue sensitivity to thyroid hormones. Progressively, the substance blunts the response of various organs to thyroxin, the principal thyroid hormone, even though the thyroid gland itself continues working throughout life without much letup.

In a young animal, one unit of thyroid hormone produces one unit of biological effect. But when given to adult animals, the same hormone unit calls forth only about one-third or even as little as one-tenth of the biological reaction. But surgical removal of the pituitary, Denckla found, restores the physiological effect in adult animals to its youthful value, or at least to 80 or 90 percent of that value. For instance, protective immune cells called phagocytes, which clear infections, decline in old rats to one-sixth their original number. By removing the pituitary and giving the animals thyroxin, Denckla gets the level back up to five and a half times its original level.

The recovery lasts indefinitely. Naturally, the animal misses the pituitary. Some bodily functions depend primarily on thyroxin and therefore can be restored fully by giving the animal thyroid hormones.

However, most functions in the body need two or three hormones, some as many as nine. Thus removing the pituitary and restoring some of the physiological functions in old animals has not yet prolonged their lives, but Denckla is hopeful.

> The pituitary controls 30 hormones in the body. And we are giving back two or three. An animal without a pituitary is a sick animal. My analogy to what we are doing is fixing a carburetor on a car but at the same time giving the car four flat tires. You're not going to drive off. But as we get more sophisticated and learn what to replace, we'll be in good shape.

Denckla has been doing more than just guessing about the existence of the death hormone. Two years ago he managed to isolate a crude extract from bovine pituitaries of what he calls DECO (decreasing oxygen consumption factor). Its effect on animal tissue matched Denckla's expectations: it blocked the effects of thyroxin on the receptors on the cell's surface. But the substance subsequently lost its potency and Denckla is engaged in a renewed effort to purify the mysterious hormone. The next step would be to design a proper antidote—a revolutionary new antiaging pill—that would block the effects of the death hormone to prolong life significantly.

Denckla's research finally explains why the lives of rats in underfeeding experiments like McCay's are prolonged only if the rodents are placed on the diet before puberty. The stretching out of the animals' growth apparently slows the synthesis and release of the death hormone.

"If we can reproduce the physiological competence of a ten-year-old—when man is at his healthiest—your expected lifespan will reach 600 years," says Denckla. "That's what we'll be dealing with in the next century."

Even if such a revolutionary event takes place one day, what it would do to the human species might be a problem. Species survive and evolve through new combinations of genes that express themselves in their offspring. It is critical for a species to produce as many new "experiments" within a relatively short time as possible. The species that survives in a changing environment is one that has the largest total population or the largest turnover or both. Yet there may be hope for man in the fact that giant tortoises live hundreds of years and their species survives.

It might be more sobering to contemplate the consequences of such life extension on women. Do we want millions of six-hundred-year-old widows who have outlived their husbands?

Although the intrinsic life-span of men and women theoretically should be the same, modern medicine has brought out some differences that favor women so that at birth females in the United States today can expect to outlive males by nearly eight years. Testosterone is believed to exercise a life-shortening effect on the male, whereas estrogen may give some women protection against heart disease before—and after—menopause. As Denckla notes, the incidence of hypertension is the same in both men and women, but its severity is always worse in men. A life-prolongation pill presumably would not alter the male–female life expectancy ratio.

Females of other species also hold an advantage over males, as this table shows:

SEX DIFFERENCES IN LIFE-SPAN

	Male	*Female*
White rat (average)	712 days	773 days
Black widow spider	100 days	271 days
Mealworm	60 days	111 days
Fruit fly	31 days	33 days
Housefly	18 days	30 days

If scientists succeed in increasing the life-span, the social problems involved would demand revision of all sorts of habits, customs, and laws. Would a marriage last four hundred years? Or would it be more desirable to have people get divorced and seek a new partner after a set time? And what about children—would women's child bearing span a two-hundred-year period? If that turned out to be the case, the globe would soon have to be evacuated. On the other hand, if you lived six hundred years, you could start on a trip to another galaxy as a child, and with appropriately fast propulsion, get there by middle age.

If a life-prolongation pill were invented, say, four hundred years ago, we would find ourselves in strange company today, to say the least. Shakespeare would still be living and, presumably, writing. Mozart would still be living and writing music—or suffering because he had burned himself out. Artists would continue to develop and perfect their techniques. The fantastic possibility of producing thinkers like Einstein who could live to be six hundred would outweigh many of the negative aspects of extending the life-span.

EPILOGUE

The Future of Mood Control

I foresee the day when we shall have the means and therefore, inevitably, the temptation, to manipulate the behavior and the intellectual functioning of all people through environmental and biochemical manipulation of the brain.

David Krech, a pioneering experimental psychologist at the University of California's Berkeley campus, made that prediction a decade ago. He said that such an ability to control moods and minds would come within five to ten years. Seldom has a more accurate forecast been made.

The capability to control emotions and behavior is already here. The big question is just how far we want to carry behavior and mood control with drugs.

Even some proponents of mood drugs abhor the idea of a happiness pill, yet at the same time they argue that it is just as important to probe and to determine the biochemical underpinnings of happiness and fulfillment as it is to determine the biochemistry of depression and schizophrenia.

There are obvious opportunities for misuse of behavior control with drugs. Consider what can happen when a program in mood control such as the ones administered by the U.S. military and the Central Intelligence Agency get out of hand. Although the events took place in the 1950s and 1960s, details are still trickling in today.

The horrors that ensued reflect little credit on the CIA or the military, even if they were operating under the impression that the Soviets had spurted ahead in mind control with drugs. In the CIA and military experiments, LSD was slipped to people in liquor and water without their knowledge—including, incredibly, unsuspecting patrons of bars in New York City and San Francisco. As a result of these tests a number of people died.

One of the most notable cases involved Dr. Frank C. Olson, a civilian chemist employed in secret drug research by the U.S. Army. In the early 1950s the CIA collaborated with the army on research involving new hallucinogenic chemicals. From time to time, groups of chemists from the CIA and the army's Fort Detrick in Frederick, Maryland, would meet in secluded settings, where they would live together for two or three days, discussing past progress and future needs.

One such meeting began on Thursday, November 19, 1953, in a lodge at the remote Deep Creek Lake in Maryland. Seven members of Olson's group and three CIA men attended the meeting. From time to time these men had kicked around the idea of administering LSD and other hallucinogens to unsuspecting people. They had agreed that a "blind" experiment would be useful but they (at least the army participants) did not consider administering hallucinogens to themselves. Little did they know that their "friends" from the CIA would surreptitiously slip the drug into their drinks. On that evening of November 18 eight of the men sipped afterdinner drinks they had poured from a bottle of Cointreau into which the CIA operatives had slipped an unknown dose of LSD. Two of the army men didn't drink, one because he was a nondrinker, the other because of heart trouble. The men who did drink were told twenty minutes after they had consumed the liquor laced with LSD that they had received the drug. By that time they had become boisterous and couldn't carry on a coherent conversation. They soon decided to go to bed. Nothing untoward seemed to happen to them immediately, except for periods of wakefulness. Aside from some evidence of fatigue, they seemed to be all right the next morning. There had been no doctors or other medical personnel in attendance during the tests. The senior CIA official present, who had informed the participants of their involuntary ingestion of LSD, was a chemist, Dr. Sidney Gottlieb, chief of the chemical division of the CIA's technical services staff.

On Monday morning, November 23, there was a sign, however, that something had gone drastically wrong in the experiment. Dr. Olson came to work that morning in a black mood. When his good friend and superior Lt. Col. Vincent Ruwet arrived at seven thirty that morning, he found Olson in an agitated state very unlike his normal cheerful self. Olson began by asking Ruwet whether Ruwet should fire him or whether Olson should resign. Perplexed, for Olson was an outstanding scientist, Ruwet asked why.

Olson replied that he felt worthless. Ruwet assured him that it wasn't so, that Olson had performed well on the test (Olson feared he had failed it) and that there was no reason for him to feel as he did. Olson seemed greatly reassured.

Olson had been working under a lot of pressure but had never before acted as he did that morning. His work was extremely exacting and definitely hazardous in a technical sense. He had to work under severe security restrictions under which it was necessary to conceal the true nature of his activities even from the other divisions on the base. He could not discuss his research with anyone except perhaps six to eight immediate associates. On occasion, security restrictions became so tight that he was at liberty to discuss certain information with only one other person at his research facility. But Olson appeared to bear these various security burdens well. His friends and colleagues knew him as an invariably cheerful and optimistic man, eager to spring to the aid of friends or even strangers in trouble.

Olson did suffer from a duodenal ulcer, but this didn't interfere with his work. Occasionally, he would tell his wife and friends that he should not be drawing retirement pay from the army (his ulcer had led to early retirement) because he felt he really didn't deserve to be paid for the ailment. Otherwise, Olson never showed any signs of extreme nervousness or of having an unbalanced mind.

When Olson came in looking disoriented on the following morning, Tuesday, November 24, Colonel Ruwet felt Olson needed help, so he got in touch with the CIA. They asked to have Olson at the airport as soon as possible. Ruwet went along to a New York M.D.'s office, accompanied by two CIA men. Ruwet returned home for Thanksgiving. Olson and one of the CIA operatives flew to Washington on Thursday, too, but upon arrival Olson became agitated and the two men returned to New York. Friday night, Olson called Ruwet in very good spirits and said he would see him the following morning. Olson told Ruwet he would be receiving treatment at a mental institution on the outskirts of Rockville, Maryland. What happened next understandably shocked Ruwet. At about 3:00 A.M. on Saturday, a CIA representative called Ruwet to tell him that Olson had jumped through the window of a tenth-floor room at the Statler Hilton Hotel in New York City and had killed himself.

Incredibly, only a mildly worded personal reprimand that would become part of their official files was issued to Gottlieb and two other CIA men, by Allen Dulles, the CIA director. Gottlieb destroyed a number of boxes of material relating to experiments with mind-altering drugs before his retirement from the CIA.

Other test subjects were physically forced to take hallucinogens. One, Harold Blauer, a patient at a New York City psychiatric institution, died from an apparent overdose of mescaline. He was a subject in tests conducted under a secret army contract.

Other test subjects suffered epilepsy attacks or attempted suicide after being given LSD in army experiments. One soldier hid under a barracks after being given LSD and had to be pulled out. In all, about fifteen hundred men were administered LSD and similar hallucinogens in army tests. Although long-term aftereffects in the participants were never followed up, the experiences of a few people that did come to light obviously caution against indiscriminate use of hallucinogens.

One of the more blatant cases conducted on contract for the military, with civilians as subjects—without their consent—concerns a woman named Mary Ray who worked as a research assistant at the University of Minnesota psychiatric hospital. She recalled before Senator Edward Kennedy's subcommittee on administrative practice and procedure in 1975 how she took part in an LSD test in a project sponsored by the air force. The test was run by a student, without any medically qualified people around. Mrs. Ray recalled her feelings after being given an injection of LSD.

> [I] went through a state of absolute terror, panic. I started out after the injection with nausea and shaking and feeling cold and wanting to run away but not knowing from what.

> I was in a state of becoming the universe. I became objects. I was in a state of absolute terror. I looked down and saw my arms which were two rivers with black threads and they were my veins. I realized that if I tried really hard, somehow I could sever the veins and I realized even though I was not really a person that I could end all this nightmare, this hell, by cutting my veins.
>
> I concentrated on this problem for what seemed like centuries because time did not exist. It was a strange time disorder. If I had some sort of sharp instrument and if I were alone, I could have killed myself. And no one seemed to know how to handle the situation. No one seemed to know what to do. It seemed like kids playing scientists.
>
> I remember one girl of 17 who definitely didn't want to be part of the experiment. I saw her as they were taking her in and she said she won't go, and they said, "Yes, you will," and she said, "Don't take me back to that hell," which makes me think she had a previous experience. They told her that she had no choice.
>
> I went back about an hour or two later and she was totally disintegrated. Before that she was a very normal-appearing person. She was attractive and talkative. But afterward she was just a mess. She was taken back to the ward and for four days she was mute, you couldn't get through to her in any way.

Of herself Mrs. Ray said: "Before this I was quite a relaxed person despite a rather traumatic life, and right after that, starting the date I got the LSD, I've been overwhelmed, flooded with anxiety almost 24 hours a day. It has never changed, and this is over nine years ago." She spoke of experiencing flashbacks, "a feeling of going back to that terrible world."

Shulgin and other designers of the new mood-influencing drugs are carefully trying to avoid such side effects in their new medications. They do this in part through planned design of the drugs to make them fit specific receptors in the brain.

But no man-made drug can be made absolutely free of side effects. In Arnold Mandell's lab, for instance, scientists recently discovered some previously unknown effects of a derivative of amphetamine that was being marketed as a weight-reducing agent without the side effects of amphetamine. Having found that the drug destroys certain cells in brains of rats, Mandell's associates quickly notified the manufacturer.

The safest source of mind-influencing drugs is thus likely to be not synthetic chemistry but the human brain itself—analogues of neurotransmitters and those remarkable neuropeptides.

Whatever the source of the first mood-control drug, it will be extraordinarily difficult to keep it under lock and key. "We have to recognize the fact that we are drug users," says Shulgin. "Let's evaluate the safety of the new drugs before they appear like mushrooms."

Statistics show that an astounding one-quarter of all prescriptions written today are for psychotropic drugs—*not* to treat psychotic or severely depressed patients but relatively normal or mildly neurotic individuals who show symptoms of anxiety, tension, insomnia, slight depression, and other types of mood disturbances often associated with life in modern society. Interestingly, the single most prescribed drug, accounting for seventeen of those twenty-five percentage points in recent years, has been chlordiazepoxide, better known as Librium.

Accordingly, anyone who thinks that promising new mood-control drugs can long be kept under wraps is deluding himself. Nearly one out of five Americans frequently uses a mood-influencing drug already, with women outnumbering men two to one.

Shulgin's own experience provides an example of how a new drug can leak from a lab. In the early 1960s, Shulgin synthesized a hallucinogenic agent one hundred times more potent than mescaline. He was seeking drugs that would clarify the relationship between biogenic amines and psychoses. Unknown to him, however, the drug, known as STP, went "commercial" in the underground drug culture, where it caught on big.

Similarly, there is no way of suppressing research on mind-influencing drugs, even if a big shadow might have been cast over such research as a result of those revelations about military and CIA misuse of mind drugs. Although the Food and Drug Administration makes it difficult to experiment with such drugs on humans, it can't stop individual researchers from trying the drugs on themselves and their friends who might volunteer. Says one scientist, "A tremendous number of researchers are experimenting with Shulgin-type drugs."

Some psychiatrists who use biochemicals think that the time has come to extend the use of existing drugs. For instance, Arnold Mandell not long ago called on fellow psychiatrists to "have the courage to develop a new vocabulary, a new set of professional goals and values along with our awareness of the subtle but pervasive effects of drugs on many if not all aspects of personality."

Mandell argues that the time has come to broaden the categories of depression, that if tricyclics, for instance, help in such syndromes as fear of interpersonal confrontations, ulcers, and so on, then they should be given to appropriate patients for those reasons.

Furthermore, with the growing numbers of elderly, some psychiatrists see the need, even a moral obligation, to supply the depressed and lonely aging (as well as people confined to wheelchairs and others without prospects of experiencing "kicks" from normal daily living) with mood-enhancing drugs.

The idea, concedes one of its principal proponents, Heinz Lehman of McGill University, "goes against the grain of everything." The teaching that doctors and psychiatrists get is that

> you age gracefully, there is nothing we can do about these problems. Aging isn't the same thing as some of the depressions we see in other people. But that's just the point, why should we accept aging? But it is indecent, or ridiculous—in the accepted view—to want to do anything about it.
>
> It just hasn't occurred to most people that the equation isn't inevitability and aging, but inevitability and death. Death can't be prevented but much of aging could be. Death isn't the same thing as aging. And the other thing that hasn't occurred to them is that while they all complain about the high incidence of depression in their patients, they don't realize that in these old people some of the depressions can be prevented. Just look at the sources of gratification that all of us have, which to these people are not available, recreation and such. That's what keeps us non-depressed.

Some of the fear in developing such drugs is that they will get into the wrong hands, be stolen from hospitals, drugstores, and so on. "People worry it would get all over the place," Lehman explains. "People would just take nice 'trips' and not do any work anymore. It would have to be controlled, but that's a technical inconvenience. They control morphine pretty well now. They accept morphine for a couple of months, for a dying cancer patient but they won't accept it for these others. Every drop of morphine is accounted for."

However, even such strong proponents of mood control with drugs as Mandell and Shulgin don't see the use of drugs as the sole means of enhancing feelings and emotions, at least in normal, healthy people. "A drug is merely a very fast, very accessible catalyst," says Shulgin. "A drug does nothing but catalyze what can be catalyzed in many other ways."

Mandell speaks enthusiastically of the euphoria that a long-distance runner experiences. And recent research at Purdue University supports the idea that rigorous physical exercise can do wonders not only for the body but for the mind, too. The Purdue researchers took sixty middle-aged staff and faculty members, all relatively unfit and almost all of whom led sedentary lives, working at their desks from eight to five. They put the men through four months of strenuous exercise.

Aside from the expected improvements in physical fitness the men also showed clear personality changes. They became more open, extroverted, and stopped complaining about physical ailments, real or imagined. Some even reported improvements in vision and hearing.

These experiments confirmed what some laymen have always known, that exercise can improve the state of one's mind. For one thing, exercise increases blood circulation to the brain, boosting the amount of glucose, which is essential to the brain's nutrition. Among other things, this prevents the craving for sweets. Exercise also appears to shift hormonal and neurotransmitter balance subtly in a beneficial direction. People who exercise tend to worry less.

Another prominent brain researcher and educator, James McGaugh of the University of California at Irvine, has, despite his pioneering work on memory-enhancing drugs, reservations about their widespread use on normal people.

On the one hand, McGaugh says that treatments for senility, mental retardation, and brain damage are clearly needed. But he also feels that there should be serious reservations about developing drugs and other treatments to be used as neurobiological aids to the education of people who do not have disorders of learning and memory.

"We've all come to accept the use of drugs as aids to daily living," McGaugh told a session at a recent annual meeting of the American Association for the Advancement of Science. "It would, I believe, be quite easy for us to accept the view that pills for improving learning and memory should be routinely taken along with vitamins, aspirin, and various patent medicines."

McGaugh feels, however, that most of the learning and remembering that we engage in does not need to be aided with drugs. He fears that such treatments could become substitutes for other conditions that aid education, that memory and learning pills would become a lazy child's or adult's crutch or shortcut. McGaugh points out that laboratory studies show that, though animals can learn more readily when given certain drugs, the same learning can be produced in the animals by giving them more training. Adds McGaugh: "The drugs don't do anything that cannot be done by providing more experience. Learning is often poor simply because the teaching or training procedures are not optimal."

An interesting problem is bound to arise when a memory pill becomes available. Will children who use it have an unfair advantage over those who don't? Parents have already objected to the use of calculators in the classroom, but the use of a memory pill would be even more difficult to control. However, if such a memory pill reduced or eliminated senile dementia in the aged it would be hard to argue against its use.

In preparing for a new "choose-your-mood" society, we should not underestimate the power of the human mind. An inner calm and courage can often be the best medicine for good mental health. People can think themselves sick and literally worry themselves to death. They can also think themselves well, treating disease through the power of the mind. An estimated 70 percent of illnesses are brought on by stress and thinking oneself sick.

Among other things, emotions heighten the galvanic potential in the skin. If a person could lower it with impulses from the brain, he could control moods, channeling them into pleasurable, beneficial directions. Medicine would thus gain a new weapon for the organism to deal with stress—without drugs and their side effects, without outside help, relying only on a person's inner strength.

Simple meditation can do wonders for body and mind. The techniques of achieving a higher consciousness through a fully rested and relaxed body and a fully awake and relaxed mind vary, but the result is the same. Some practitioners of yoga in India arrive at the relaxed state through strenuous physical exercise, some focus on mental concentration or contemplation, and others try to control a particular bodily function, such as the respiratory rate.

One widely practiced and easily learned yoga technique, transcendental meditation (TM), has been popularized in the United States by Maharishi Mahesh Yogi. In this approach the subject sits in a comfortable chair and perceives a sound or thought. Without concentrating specifically on this cue, the TM practitioner allows his mind to float around it. Interestingly, even this readily acquired technique places its practitioners in a relaxed state very close to that attained by Zen Buddhist monks and Indian yogis who spend years and decades mastering the meditative state.

EEG patterns during meditation show that the alpha waves—brain waves that become prominent when a person is thoroughly relaxed—of TM practitioners resemble the EEG patterns recorded in yogi and expert Zen meditators. Other physiological correlates of the TM state hint at the power of mind over moods: oxygen consumption drops significantly and output of carbon dioxide is decreased, indicating a slowing of metabolism. Similarly, the level of lactate in the blood drops. This is bound to have a beneficial effect, since patients with an anxiety neurosis display a large rise in blood lactate when they find themselves in stress situations. Infusions of lactate can also produce symptoms of anxiety in normal subjects. In transcendental meditators, low lactate is associated with low blood pressure. All in all, this pattern of changes—induced without any calming drugs—is a kind of relax-and-enjoy counterpart to the famous fight-or-flight syndrome, in which the nervous system mobilizes physiological responses, increasing blood pressure, heart rate, and flow of blood to the muscles, as well as oxygen consumption.

In the view of many scientists, the fight-or-flight response to threats, real or imagined, undoubtedly performed a highly useful function in man's early history. But in today's world it may have largely outlived its usefulness. In fact, stimulation of this defense-alarm mechanism by frequent stresses in the environment is what is believed to be largely responsible for the high incidence of high blood pressure and other degenerative diseases and mental ailments that mark life in our society. Conversely, the practice of meditation could serve as a route to better health.

Biofeedback, the possibility of enhanced self-control, is exciting but scientifically unproven for the most part and is vastly oversold to the public by the mass media. To cash in on the tremendous public interest in the field, entrepreneurs have jumped into the field to sell poor-quality equipment that they claim enhances alpha rhythms and produces other biofeedback benefits. Most specialists doubt that such equipment can in fact generate the electronic enlightenment advertised, though some feel that the equipment may be interesting to experiment with.

The full potential of the human brain remains to be delineated. Natalie Bekhterev, director of the Moscow Institute of Experimental Medicine, wrote recently:

> You can train a hand but muscle power is limited. The heart has similar limits to overload. The brain has no such shortcomings. When we become distracted from our main task at hand, the brain cells responsible for it don't simply rest. Something so far unexplained happens: the thoughts, so to speak, "ripen" during that time. The more varied our interests the better, since ever larger portions of the brain get involved and the brain acquires new capabilities.

Memory, in particular, improves the more we learn, and almost everyone could benefit from an improved memory. In fact, it's often a phenomenal memory that makes a person highly successful in his chosen field. For instance, Isaac Asimov, scientist and author of nearly 120 books, has such a fantastic memory that he seldom has to do research for his books—and they have ranged from an interpretation of the Bible to a book about photosynthesis.

For the rest of us, whose memories aren't quite as good, there are proven techniques of expanding our capacities to remember. Mnemonists, specialists who teach how memory can be improved, long ago discovered aids to better remembering. In general, memory is greatly enhanced by improving the organization of the information at the time it is stored. Seven seems to be the magic number for most people for remembering things. For example, most people can remember strings of numbers in a row, but most have difficulty remembering more than seven.

There is a way of overcoming that limit, however, by "chunking," or grouping together several items. They can then be committed to memory as a block. When Alexander Solzhenitsyn, the exiled Soviet author, was in a concentration camp, without access to writing materials, he composed and memorized a poem of 10,000 lines. He was helped by some fellow prisoners, Roman Catholics, who made beads for him to aid in the task of memorizing.

The science of mood control traces its roots to phrenology, the now discredited attempt to tie bumps on the skull with emotions and psychological faculties such as physical love, aggressiveness, self-esteem, intelligence, and so on.

The modern science of mood control seeks instead to relate the functions of the brain's anatomical organization to those of chemical "colors," the mixtures of neurotransmitters and neuropeptides. Mood control thus seeks to combine chemical specificity with anatomical specificity, not outside the skull but inside it. The new science of mood control is, in short, after nothing less than a "mood map" that will allow a degree of precision in manipulation undreamed of by the phrenologists or even by modern scientists just a few years ago. The weapons of manipulation are the new drugs, diets, meditation, and other means such as biofeedback and exercise.

Separating these components of mind and mood control doesn't make sense. With a vitamin B deficiency, for instance, we get a memory loss because vitamin components act as coenzymes in the synthesis of RNA in the brain, which is needed for memory consolidation.

The close link between these seemingly diverse elements calls for a sensitive, total approach to good mental health. It's not only the proper vitamins that our bodies and minds need but also exercise, sunlight, rest, and the plain equanimity of spirit. The new mood and mind-influencing drugs should not become a permanent crutch for healthy, normal people but only an occasional means to extend our natural capabilities. Just as the early tranquilizers and antidepressants served to pinpoint the biochemical pathways of mental anguish and led to their amelioration, so should the new mood-influencing drugs point the way to enhanced emotions and sharpened capabilities.

But if the use of mood-control drugs so far has already produced a raging controversy, one can easily imagine the explosive impact of such novel developments as that ultimate aphrodisiac from the brain. Guided into constructive channels, however, these remarkable advances in mood and mind control can lead man to a happier, fuller life.

Index

1.45

467

47